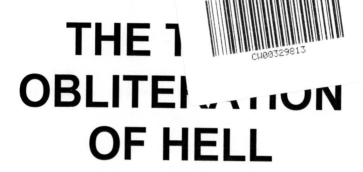

THE TOTAL OBLITERATION OF HELL

Frank Hayward

chipmunkapublishing
the mental health publisher
empowering people with psychosis

Frank Hayward

Published by
Chipmunkapublishing
PO Box 6872
Brentwood
Essex CM13 1ZT
United Kingdom

http://www.chipmunkapublishing.com

Chipmunkapublishing gratefully acknowledge the support of Arts Council England.

ACKNOWLEDGEMENTS

I would like to thank Anne Agudo for proofreading the manuscript and for encouraging me to be critical of my work; my former Community Mental Health Nurse Nick for suggesting that I divide the book into headed chapters; my brother Peter for his assistance with the word processor, and Lola Jimenez for any inadvertent contribution she may have made towards driving me crazy and thus to giving me something to write about and saving me from the conventional life I had feared I would feel obliged to embrace.

For Kevin – may he find the peace that passeth all understanding.

Frank Hayward

The Total Obliteration Of Hell

Introduction

My present life, so I'm told, and maybe it's my first?, began in Chase Farm Hospital, London, England. I have a picture in my mind's eye of sunlight on a wall that seems to attribute itself to my first days in the hospital, but it is probably just a fantasy that I've built up since, for I have no other 'memories' of the first three or four years of my life. – And it was to Chase Farm that I was 'recalled' a quarter of a century later, though at the time I barely recognized it as a hospital, besides which I was sure I'd died, and had moved to some other plane of consciousness.

I have little idea where to begin when speaking of the development of my insanity, partly because I am, even now, pretty much in the dark as to the time of, and reasons for, its inception, and partly since many of the people I had come to know during the twenty five years preceding my admission to the Psychiatric Unit were of the unequivocal opinion that I had 'always' been 'a little touched'. So I'll not try to trace the evolution of what 'blossomed' into a raging disorder of the mind, but instead simply begin at the point at which I myself became aware of a distinct change in my perceptions, or rather, a change in the feel and appearance of the world I perceived as being external to me.

Frank Hayward

The Total Obliteration Of Hell

PART 1:1985

The journey to Utrecht

On about February 10th 1985, my father drove me to my college in his Volkswagen Golf. It was a crisp, clear morning, and I was excited about the field course to Utrecht in the Netherlands upon which myself and my fellow students (on the 'Town and Country Planning' specialization of a B.A. Social Science degree) were due to embark that morning, along with members of staff that included my tutor Angela. Having deposited my bag in the corridor in which students and luggage were accumulating prior to boarding the coach, I went and banged on the keys of the piano on the stage in the main hall for a few minutes, and then returned to the corridor, studiously avoiding the voluptuous Amy Franks with my eyes. Once on the coach, I read a long article on the husbandry of Mediterranean tortoises in the herpetological magazine that I'd received in the post that morning, and also read; or reread?, the disaffected letter from my Spanish pen-friend Lola, which had also arrived that day. I was full of 'eager' indignation at her suggestion that maybe she should stop writing to me and, full of my 'great love', endeavoured to devise a means of telling her off.

We were now well into the journey to Harwich, where we were to board the ferry for the continent, and I was in a fine, ebullient mood. I suppose that the thought of exotic, drunken nights, with the 'forbidden' temptation of Amy likely to be only a few yards away, had got me high. It was at this point that the coach windscreen shattered. As far as I can recall, this curious incident, although a talking point for the next few minutes, aroused little reaction, and, as far as I was concerned, merely served as an excuse to try out my Russian style hat on account of the draught.

I don't recall us changing coach (we may have done); neither do I remember boarding the ferry, but the trip across the water stands out in my mind, primarily for the profound effect that I gauged the film that I spent two hours of the crossing watching, had on me, an effect by no means lessened by the unexpected, but seemingly appropriate, arrival of Amy in the cinema shortly after I'd taken my seat. The film; 'The Natural', engaged my imagination in what might on reflection be described as the beginning of a heady descent into a world of delusion, and I proceeded to attach an incredible amount of significance to certain scenes, and somehow wove my own story of absolute good and total evil. Indeed, even the title 'The Natural' became imbued with mystical meaning in my eyes and, by the time the film ended, I was quite decided that Robert Redford, who played the central character, was possessed of most extraordinary psychic gifts. As I left the cinema, I was seriously contemplating asking Amy if I could buy her a drink, but she was with someone and I let her be. – I spent the remainder of the ferry trip in the bar, laughing and joking with some of the other students, including Joseph from Zimbabwe.

The Total Obliteration Of Hell

Having crossed the channel, there are two things that stick in my mind about the remainder of the journey; namely, being ushered into a building somewhat akin to an aircraft hangar and thinking that maybe we'd be searched, and perhaps even shot!, and standing in a shopping mall, where Amy dared me to try and make myself understood in order to buy a cigarette lighter.

Frank Hayward

The field course

The next thing that I remember distinctly occurred after our arrival in Utrecht (I'm not sure that I was particularly aware that we were in Utrecht), when the question of who was going to share a room with whom was being discussed. I think that I made light of this matter; I can't remember precisely what I said, but it was along the lines of, 'who would be prepared to tolerate sharing a room with me?' I don't remember anything else that I'm sure occurred on the day of our journey and arrival, and indeed, I would find it impossible without discovering an old diary (and I'm not sure that I kept one) to outline the events of the following days in any accurate kind of chronological sequence. The only thing of which I am fairly certain in terms of the order of events is that I spent most, if not all, the evenings, in the two bars contained within the building in which we were staying. But I have many abiding, albeit blurry-edged, memories of the week, which I will try to relate to the best of my ability, as soon as I have briefly mentioned what is perhaps a rather obvious potential pitfall.

In the same way that it is, as I have already suggested, hard to pinpoint the events surrounding the early development of my 'mental condition', neither is it an easy matter to trace a sequence of events that charts the deterioration of my health during our week in Holland. And the fact that that very deterioration was affecting me obviously exacerbates the difficulty. To make an analogy, it is

The Total Obliteration Of Hell

like trying to develop clear pictures from a film that has been used in a camera with a damaged lens. But perhaps I am overstating the problem, or simply missing the point of the exercise, which might be described as the conveying of an impression of what it's like to be unbalanced in one's mind from the point of view of someone who has been. 'We' will just have to see whether what develops makes some sort of sense, or appears as no more than a list of strange incidents with nothing more in common than their unusual nature.

Not long before journeying to Holland – maybe a few months, perhaps a year – I had become interested in the oriental religious philosophy of Taoism, and had somehow cottoned on (not necessarily justifiably) to the idea that, basically, the notion of planning anything was foolish, because life was to be lived spontaneously, without recourse to such things as the intellectual prescriptions of the Social Sciences. And adding to this the facts that I was completely in love with my supposed wisdom, which I considered to be superior to that of my peers and the staff at the college (perhaps by way of reaction to a sense of rejection?), and that, as a consequence of this, I felt isolated from my fellow man, plus a desperate lonely yearning to relate to somebody, one has the recipe for the resultant fantasy: - I decided almost straightaway that the Dutch were a living embodiment of the way the world ought to be, at least in terms of getting their country 'planned'. (I'm not sure what, if any, evidence I can cite for forming my stubborn conclusion that the inhabitants of this nation could 'see beyond the sham of planning'; perhaps my head was turned by the (debatably) cool, quietly spoken manner of the Dutch planners with whom we met, or the reserved curiosity they may have quite innocently displayed towards members of another white race?) And I was just as sure that these 'amazing' people had a highly advanced telepathic ability. But investing the Dutch, and specifically these planners, with great insight into how life ought to be lived and the ability to read thoughts was also slightly disconcerting, since I was aware that they too might not be my allies. Whether this was reflective of a paranoia that I was biologically developing, or is a form of mistrust that is a natural consequence of isolation and a wish to meet 'genuinely intelligent life forms' I don't know, but, if the latter, then maybe the likely development of paranoia, or of a particular form of paranoia, can be predicted, and thus avoided by early intervention. But further consideration of this is outside the scope of this small volume.

As I have suggested, I quickly formed some very definite ideas concerning the psychological cum spiritual nature of the Dutch people. It occurs to me that perhaps I was, subconsciously, or even to an extent consciously, influenced into my dogmatic and sweepingly generalized opinions by something I'd read not long before in Shirley MacLaine's autobiographical 'Out On A Limb', in which Ms. MacLaine refers to a spiritual medium who, although in fact Swedish, may have been remembered by me as having been Dutch. There is, admittedly, no suggestion in Shirley's book that

The Total Obliteration Of Hell

the Dutch (or rather the Swedish) are any more psychic than any other nationality, but at least the germ of my idea can be seen. – Anyway, having decided that the Dutch were perfectly well aware that planning was a fundamental waste of time, and that therefore, our meetings with these continental 'planners' were simply cosmetic exercises, in which our party was simply being humoured and given the appropriate 'bumf', and that what was really going on was being conveyed only by the odd discreet glance, which only I was capable of understanding, I suppose that I felt that there was very little point in my paying much attention to the information they were diplomatically disseminating. At any rate, whatever the reason; and maybe my ability to concentrate was already impaired by the maelstrom of my thoughts, I did indeed pay very little heed to what was going on, and instead, devoted my attention to my obsession with my 'glorious love' for my Lola. I am not sure whether I actually wrote anything on this subject, although I had been spending time during planning lectures prior to the Dutch trip writing my 'masterwork'; 'The World of Lola Jimenez Part 1'. I have no record of which I am aware of any letters penned during the field course to my 'girlfriend of a lifetime', chastising her for suggesting the possibility that our correspondence should cease, and as to whether I added to the material of my book about her (this was really mostly about my hang ups) I cannot be certain, since the rough drafts that I possess are not dated as a letter would be: - it seems likely that I scribbled something down. But I am in no doubt that Lola's letter, and how I would respond to it, preyed rapaciously on my mind. What I find more difficult to remember is whether I was conscious of any consequent mental anguish which might have catalyzed my decline into the hell into which I subsequently found I had fallen. At all events, I began to drink, and whether or not because of this, began to lose my limited awareness of the behaviour of those around me, to the extent that I became oblivious to the usual psychological landmarks by which most of us in ordinary health order our lives. Under more normal circumstances, many of my actions, had I performed them, would have caused me acute embarrassment, and shame and anxiety that corresponded to my longstanding fear of authority. As it was, I was past caring about 'appropriate social behaviour', and completely given over to the intensity of hitherto undreamed of sensation. This may suggest that I had lapsed into the taking of illicit drugs, and I have often wondered whether I did indeed get hold of some substance about which I have subsequently forgotten, or even whether something that I ate or drank had been laced with some 'mind expanding' drug. However, to the best of my knowledge, all I had, besides alcohol and 'regular' cigarettes was a modest amount of marijuana, and this had not, on the rare occasions upon which I'd previously smoked it, produced any dramatic 'altered state'. (I daresay that the dope may have played a part though; i.e., assuming that I was more susceptible than usual to anything out of the ordinary).

As I have already indicated, one of my then current preoccupations involved Amy; a playful, feisty (to

The Total Obliteration Of Hell

use what is now the fashionable term) blonde from the West Country, with a face and body made to flaunt. We'd had a stormy acquaintance over the past couple of years; I'd always found her highly sexually provocative, and had, true to type, written her absurd letters, and sabotaged (deliberately?) any remote chance of getting to know her more intimately. But then after all, I'd made a vow to myself the previous year that I would be faithful to Lola, whether Lola cared or did not. However, as the Dutch field course had approached, my frustration at spurning the favour I imaginatively felt that Amy had been showing me had intensified, and I had increasingly been feeling that, should the opportunity present itself, there would be no way that I would try, or even wish to try, to contain my lust. Perhaps it is fortunate that, in the event, my mushrooming incoherence, and equally heavy preoccupation with my 'journey into the world of the spirit', effectively neutralized my libido and, I suspect, acted as a strong deterrent to any possible interest on her part. But that is not to say that I was unaware of her presence. But it wasn't just her visible proximity that stimulated me.

There was an upright piano in the bar that we had been invited to utilize, and manage, as guests, and (and this will hopefully serve as a fitting example of the depths of delusive fantasy I'd now reached) I was somehow quite certain that Amy responded, probably without realizing it, to the sequence of notes from 'Close Encounters Of The Third Kind', by appearing whenever I played it. I suppose that it is possible that, by pure coincidence, she'd happened to walk into the bar just after I'd played this motif (or call sign as I regarded it) on one occasion, and maybe this had even happened more than once; whatever, I was 'captured' by my belief that I had a Svengali-like power over her. I suppose that, however foolish such an idea may appear in isolation, it is perfectly consistent with the absurdly arrogant attitude of a man who thinks that the most desirable woman cannot resist him, notwithstanding any amount of evidence to the contrary. I noticed sometimes (maybe it was only once) that she came and stood alone at the bar not far from where I was ensconced. And of course I thought it significant. And of course I ignored her.

Our party had been split into groups for the purpose of visiting different locations, and I, to my chagrin, was not in the same one as Amy. However, one morning, I was so completely unmotivated that I simply couldn't be bothered to be ready in time to leave with the section of the student body to which I'd been assigned, and found myself tagging along with her 'set'. As I recall, the day that I switched groups, we met with a Dutch Moluccan. I have no clear recollection of the substance of his conversation, though I believe that it concerned the situation of ethnic minorities in the Netherlands. What I remember more vividly is that I needed to leave the room and smoke a cigarette: - the first sign of the restlessness that would later plague me and render me quite incapable of staying in one place? And, as I stood in the doorway and looked at everyone, it seemed to me that theirs was a very different world from mine, and very far away. The only other thing that I remember for certain about that day is hanging around after the talk in order to get close to Amy. I doubt if any words were exchanged.

Although I wasn't hallucinating exactly, I was aware of transient shapes and light when gazing at supposedly plain and solid objects such as walls, as if I had a kind of 'second sight', by which all that I mean to say is that I felt that 'invisible spirit forms' were now accessible to my vision. And I'd also developed the notion that I could detect what one might call 'sites of spiritual energy'. The verbalizing of these impressions does not really bring out the vague, elusive, and ever changing feelings that were hitting me. At one point we were in a 'courtyard'?, and I was sure that the 'Lost Ark of the Covenant' was close at hand. (See later for more of my 'Indiana Jones' fantasies.)

I had been a vegetarian for about six months prior to going to Holland, and an appropriate diet had been requested for me. However, as the week progressed, I began to care less what I ate, perhaps partly because I wasn't convinced that the supposedly suitable comestibles I was being offered were in fact free of meat; the logic being that therefore there wasn't much point in fussing. I cannot specifically recall any of the mealtime conversations, but I do remember that I sat at least once at a table with one James Stephenson, and that I was particularly attentive to whatever it was that he was talking about. I also remember one occasion on which I strolled over to where Amy had been sitting at table, and finished the glass of water that she'd left partly drunk. (I may have been hoping that someone would report my behaviour to her, and that she would be impressed.)

As I have said, there were two bars attached to where we were staying in Utrecht, and on at least one evening I paid a visit to the upstairs one (this was not I think really intended for the use of our group) and got talking, as far as I was still capable of doing so, to some of the Dutch girls there: - God only knows what about! And, although it may be an idle dream that I subsequently manufactured, my memory tells me that I engaged in a long kiss with one of the girls. I don't remember being reprimanded by her or any of the other girls for inappropriate behaviour, but I cannot imagine that it was greatly to her liking, although, for all I know, she may have encouraged me.

As the field course approached its termination, so the time was fast approaching for 'we' students to present our findings, or at least, our thoughts about what we'd experienced; ie, in relation to the course work! Accordingly, we gathered in the lecture hall, and spoke in turn in groups of two or three in front of the others. I believe that the small group to which I was assigned had been briefed by Angela, but I cannot remember if I was supposed to be a spokesperson. In the event, I found that I was far too immersed in expressing some 'deep thoughts' on a long roll of paper to pay much attention to the proceedings, which were pretty unintelligible and irrelevant anyway, or so I felt at the time. No doubt I would have liked to have 'played to the gallery', but, when it comes down to it, I was simply too far gone, and, in retrospect, I think that everyone present realized it.

Other memories of the time in Utrecht include travelling on a (public) bus and having no idea where to get off in order to return to base (fortunately I realized in time that some of the other students were also on board, and so followed them), and standing by a building from which the sound of a siren or burglar alarm was issuing and willing the noise to cease by a concentrated effort of mind. And then there was the then current pop song 'Black Man Ray', which convinced me that one of the students was thoroughly evil. I remember watching him kicking a football about in the garden behind the house in which we were staying, and thinking that it was the action of someone who was up to no good.

Frank Hayward

Being naughty in Amsterdam

There was still one full day left before we were due to catch the overnight ferry back to England, and it had been arranged that we would spend it sightseeing in Amsterdam. This had been planned before we left England, and I'd had it in mind that I would go and visit the zoo. However, by the time the day arrived, I don't think I cared very much one way or the other and, when our train reached Amsterdam (I believe that we went by rail), I don't think that the by now phenomenal task of finding it on a city plan interested me very much and, leaving the other students to do as they saw fit, I wandered aimlessly about the square in front of the station. I recollect that there was someone in the square playing a guitar and, in pausing briefly to listen, I emptied my pockets onto the ground in a manner that I felt befitted someone of what I considered to be my advanced spiritual development, as if to show that I was not greatly concerned about my material possessions. (It is probably nearer the truth that I couldn't find something; eg, rizla papers.) After having partaken of 'one or two' roll-ups, I couldn't think of anything else to do, and so drifted into a bar and somehow managed to obtain a drink although, as to whether I actually ordered one, or simply 'took possession' of one that had apparently been left there, I'm not quite sure. I don't know if I engaged in any conversation in English with any of the bar staff, or whether, if I did say something, it was understood. I don't think that I made any effort to pay for my drink, or for any that I

The Total Obliteration Of Hell

subsequently drank, and, maybe because of this, or because I kept staring (which I also only may have done), it was eventually made plain to me that I was no longer welcome there. Comparatively undaunted, I sauntered about in at least one sex shop; buying a magazine for what I considered to be a striking resemblance between a girl depicted therein engaged in an unrepeatable activity, and Amy. (I could 'actually see her wince' as 'she realized' that I was looking at 'her'.) I spent the rest of the day sitting in a seedy coffee bar; relieving my sexual frustration in public toilets, and procuring a small amount of dope from a man who approached me on the street.

At some stage in the late afternoon/early evening, it occurred to me that I'd quite forgotten the time of the train we were due to catch for the Hook of Holland and, perhaps surprisingly, bearing in mind my somewhat torpid, sensual condition, this did actually trigger a mild panic in me. It is probably just as well that fate was kind enough to reunite me with the reassembling segments of our party in good time for the off.

I showed my friend Mark the dope that I'd bought, and he had to 'shush' me, since I was speaking in rather a loud voice, and (probably) waving it around. I think that he for one had more or less given up on me by this time. During the train journey, a refreshments trolley was wheeled past, and when I saw, or heard someone mention, an egg roll, I was quite sure that it symbolized some sort of sexual perversion. But it was only once on board the ferry back to Harwich that my world really 'turned over'.

The Total Obliteration Of Hell

In a trance on the ferry

There was a small dance floor area on the ferry, and the latest chart hits were being pumped out. I was sitting with the somewhat macho Joseph above the dance floor, and I was getting a bit fed up by what I felt was his uncalled for bragging about his prowess with women. I think that he sensed my hostility. I'm not quite sure how it happened but, at some stage, a table tennis ball came into my possession, and it seemed appropriate to hasten along to the cinema area in order to show anyone who was willing to see, my 'trick' involving the ball and the screen. It is not now clear to me quite what I intended as I rushed into the auditorium (without a ticket, naturally!), but I remember that it related to the film 'The Natural' that I'd seen on the outward journey. At the end of this film, a baseball is hit way over the top of a stadium, and simply keeps on going. (I suppose on reflection I was trying to somehow confirm my own supposed psychic ability.)

Either before or after the incident with the table tennis ball, I investigated the passengers' lounge, and discovered Amy sitting quite innocently with two of the more mature male students. I sat down at a nearby table and muttered something about 'Superman': - I was still full of the notion that in spite of herself, she found me irresistible. I may also have referred to 'Helen of Troy', for I was rapidly coming to the conclusion that such was Amy's true identity. I don't believe that she spoke to me; I think that she looked mildly alarmed. I didn't stop for long; I was 'on a roll', and, once well lubricated at the bar, took to the dance floor to the strains of the 'devilish' 'Power of Love' by 'Frankie Goes To Hollywood'; a 'mega band' destined to become my imagined passport to superstardom (see later). Whilst I'd been sitting above the dance area, I'd looked at the stage, and had visualized the appearance of some or other famous rock star, and of Amy in her 'true guise' of Helen: - she would proceed to divest herself of the skimpy clothing she was wearing. Now as I danced however, it was just me, mirrored by the screen backing the dance floor; whirling and gyrating ever more rapidly, 'dazzled by my brilliance'; hypnotized perhaps? I was sweating now and, unbuttoning my shirt, slumped down amongst some 'life bags'.

I don't know for how long I lay like that; I don't think that it was a particularly long time, but I do know that I had no wish to move. After a while, some uniformed staff helped me to my feet, and, supporting me, led me away. I can't remember where I was deposited, but I do recall that at some stage later on I was lying down in the corridor between the cabins in a strange state of muted consciousness (one could I suppose call it a trance) and once again had no inclination to move. Time passed, and I became aware of the voices of some of the students, and recognized one of the lecturers. Again I was helped to my feet, and was walked to my cabin.

The Total Obliteration Of Hell

As I lay sluggishly in bed (I doubt very much that I took the trouble to undress), my thoughts passed sentence on me; I had played with knowledge and tried to be too smart, and now I was going to have to pay the price. And, as I continued in this vein, I was sure that my tutor Angela was passing this message to me telepathically. I was not sure that I could hear her voice, and I saw no vision of her face; there was just a strong sense that she was with me. After further time, it occurred to me that perhaps I was okay, but that Angela had been 'captured' by the 'Moonies'. I'm not sure if I felt that I was also undergoing brainwashing (see later). Prior to losing consciousness for the night, I have a very powerful memory of gazing into a mirror, and wondering (a), whether I could walk through it into the reflected world, and (b), whether I was already on the far side of the mirror and in a different dimension.

Apparently I was found in the toilet the following morning about half an hour after the ferry had docked. – I'm not certain how I made it through customs because I'm sure that I wasn't holding my passport, but maybe Angela or one of the other lecturers explained that I was 'not a well man'. Boarding the coach home everyone was passive and, to my mind, in a trance. I suppose that I felt that I was in a trance as well, but that, unlike the others, I was smart enough to realize it, and I felt quite alone amongst them. And the banana yellow sunlight was not the sunlight that I had known, or at least I thought not. – My conviction that I was no longer in the world that I'd known up to a week ago was clearly starting to take hold.

Amy was at the rear of the coach, and once again surrounded by the burly forms of Alan and Brian. I approached her, muttering something about a sleeping princess, and then went and took a seat further forward.

The Total Obliteration Of Hell

My return to Willow Walk.

Back in Enfield Town, people were being dropped off. Amy got out, and entered a telephone kiosk, and I got out; probably with the intention of following her, but something held me back. I believe that watching her talking made me think of the white rabbit in 'Alice in Wonderland': - I'm not sure why. – Having got my luggage, I wandered off in the vague direction of home although, in this 'strange world', I wasn't quite sure that it was the best plan. Passing shop windows, all the eyes of the pop and movie stars in the posters seemed to be gazing at me pleadingly, and I pondered the possibility that there was something that I had to do to help humanity. Leaving the town, I took a footpath for home; changed my mind, returned to the town, and then, with my mind made up as far as it could be, started again for Willow Walk, but by a more direct route beside a busy road.

A quarter of a mile further on I was intercepted by Angela and a woman who I was convinced was a spiritual medium: - her sister in fact. They offered me a lift home. I wasn't sure that I trusted their motives. (If you remember, I had come to the tentative conclusion that Angela was involved with the 'Moonies'.) However, the thought that I might be abducted was outweighed by the consideration that I wouldn't have to carry my luggage any further should I accept the lift. On arriving outside my house, Angela came to the door. She seemed a bit downcast to me, and I tried to reassure her. I believe that I said that I'd see her in two weeks' time; the significance of the two weeks is a mystery to me. (In fact, I believe that I first went inside the house and shut the door rather abruptly, and that Angela rang the doorbell, whereupon I answered the door and said my short piece about the two weeks.)

The Total Obliteration Of Hell

An unusual homecoming

At some stage during the afternoon of my return home I discovered my mother laid up in bed, with a cold sore above her upper lip that, to my mind, betrayed her true character; a monster on the scale of Hitler, whose face hers called to mind at the time. I think that I may have let this opinion slip out, but, whether I did or not, I thought that her apparent alarm reflected a realization that I'd seen 'the awful truth' about her. (In fact, what was bothering her, besides a most unpleasant leg condition and pains in her back, was the change that was evident in me, for gone was her eccentric, but loveable, son, and in his place stood a 'raving lunatic', wildly gesticulating as he uttered such phrases as 'make my day Amy!', as he visualized 'little golden sparks of Amy', or rather the sun, as she had now 'become'.)

For much of the remainder of that day I was crashed out on my bed, feeling heavy and entirely lacking in energy, and staring up at the 'lampshade goddess'; 'Mayan' from Shirley MacLaine's 'Out On A Limb', who was 'sucking out my brain'. I was tranquil; convinced that I was dying, and fantasizing about awakening in an afterlife with Lola at my bedside, she having committed suicide in sympathy with my having died of a broken heart because she'd rejected me. The sounds of the cars outside lulled me, and I imagined that when I awoke there'd be birdsong, and no more cars, and that the 'new earth' would be filled with celebration because I'd died and saved the 'sad old world'. But it wasn't to be quite as I'd hoped; not quite!

I awoke during the night and, making my way to the back half of my bedroom, discovered that one of my (pet) lizards; a 'Flying Gecko', had died. I was so sure of my powers to heal that I little doubted that I could revive it by holding it between my palms and stroking. However, when no positive result was forthcoming I soon felt foolish, and decided that I was still far too conceited, and that it would be best to live humbly and simply from now on.

Descending to the lounge, I placed the L.P. soundtrack to Spielberg's 'E.T.' on the turntable, and was struck by the seeming 'cosmic eeriness' of the opening section of side one. I'm not sure if I played any other music before returning to bed. Lola was not at my bedside the following morning, but I was not without faith; maybe she'd be waiting downstairs, or would arrive by breakfast time? The television was on in the dining room, and it seemed to me that the news was just a joke; after all, the world had surely been saved. Yes; awful news stories no longer needed to be taken seriously. But then the actress Jan Francis appeared on the screen and made an appeal about something, and I was at once no longer as sure that things really were hunky dory: - perhaps the assumption of heavenly conditions required at least one more battle? Yes; Jan was 'Gill' out of 'Narnia', and whom I'd met in Scotland in '83, and was warning me to be vigilant, and to keep the faith going in

The Total Obliteration Of Hell

'Aslan', and assuring me that she loved me like a sister.

In the sunny kitchen, my father was making an omelet, and the omelet was at once a 'golden Amy', 'making my day'. I stood dreamily by the frying pan. My father appeared to be in a foul temper, and snapped at me for not watching the pan properly. My brother Peter appeared, and flashed me the vaguest glimmer of a knowing look, and I realized (or thought I did) that I could trust him, but that my father was a 'beast', and would try his utmost to 'muck up heaven and earth'.

Frank Hayward

A walk in the park

Lola had not appeared, and I got to thinking
(perhaps because of Jan's appeal?) that maybe
she (Lola) was in great danger, and decided that I'd
better leave straightaway for Madrid. After all, I still
had about £200 in the building society. I tried to be
discreet as I rummaged about in my bag, but
suspected that I'd made my intentions obvious by
donning my 'salt and pepper' overcoat. At all
events, my father invited me for a walk in the park.

It was a sunny morning, and the ground was
streaked with snow as we made our way through
the south- eastern sector of Oakwood Park and on
into Groveland's. Although not according to plan, I
was not entirely lacking in optimism that the
opportunity to escape to the building society (and
thence the underground) would present itself and,
bearing this in mind, focussed on my heavy
breathing in the chilly air, in the belief that this
would send father into a trance: - I was sure that
this was what Aslan would do, and wasn't I in effect
trying to please the great lion? However, when our
route began to draw away from my intended
direction, I very soon decided that I'd have to make
a dash for it. But my endeavour was doomed from
the start, for as I broke into a poor attempt at a run,
a series of howls worthy of Lucifer himself issued
forth from my father and, try as I might, I felt myself
powerless to break away.

The Total Obliteration Of Hell

As we continued our walk, dad assumed a much gentler frame, and 'prattled on' about buying some mushrooms at the green. Whilst returning from the shops, I re-evaluated my position, and decided that I was going to have to have some patience if I was really going to escape from my parents; in short, I'd have to 'reconstruct them psychologically' in order to sever the ties that bound me to them. (Reflecting on this, I suppose that it could be said that there was a certain degree of astuteness to my observations; ie, my realization of the strength of my bond with my father and mother.) As far as my father was concerned, and based on the incident in Groveland's, I was reminded of the film 'Harvey', in which the character played by James Stewart relied for his peace of mind upon his sense of awareness of the presence of an 'invisible' white rabbit: - maybe dad needed me in a similar way?

In which I go indirectly to hell

Upon returning home, I sat, or stood (and probably both in turn) in the dining room, 'cosmically dancing' with my fingers, hands and arms; 'summoning E.T.'. My family was silent. Angela and Dave Jones promptly arrived, and it felt like my cue to leave.

All the way to the college I was sure that E.T. was approaching, and I believe that I felt that everything in heaven and earth would shortly be resolved. I'm not quite sure who it was that I saw at the college, but I remember that I was invited to recline on a couch. I think that my feeling was that I was being tested, and that, if I passed, I would be presented with my degree for having 'saved the world'. And I was quite expecting to see the familiar faces of all my fellow students coming to meet me. And (and I'm entirely certain of this) I thought of 'Alice in Wonderland' again, as if it related to the reality of the present. However, after a short time, and having seen no familiar faces, it was back to the car, and we were on our way to 'Chase Farm', although I'm not sure that I knew it.

Our wait in casualty presented me with a further opportunity to fantasize, and my thoughts were along the following lines, although I very much doubt that I was aware at the time of any structure or order.

The Total Obliteration Of Hell

Firstly, I had not saved the world. This was obvious because, had I done so, I'd be feeling alright, and wouldn't be in this awful place, filled with apprehension. Secondly, whatever was about to happen would unquestionably seal my fate in my afterlife: - I was now either almost dead, or dead and in a sort of limbo. And thirdly, I had to try and influence events to save my soul from falling into hell.

There were two large television screens in the waiting area, and it occurred to me that the drama about to be enacted might bear some sort of relation to what was being shown, or was about to be shown, on T.V. I am not now entirely certain as to whether the programmes seemed to be giving me clues as to how to act, or whether I just wished for 'Superman' or 'Indiana Jones' to appear but, in my troubled and somewhat restless state, time seemed to be of the essence, besides which, my brain was working overtime interpreting all the apparently strange phenomena round about me, and formulating a course of action for me to pursue.

Angela and Dave Jones were seated close by. Angela 'had become' my spiritual sister (perhaps 'Princess Leia' out of 'Star Wars'), and Dave 'was now' 'the beast' (maybe one of the Nazis from 'Raiders of the Lost Ark'). And, if I was in fact 'Indiana Jones', then Lola had to be 'Marion Ravenwood'. – Lola! My fantasy pursued the notion that perhaps, if I could make it out of this building and as far as Oakwood car park (where I'd first met Lola), I'd find that she'd be waiting. Continuing along this line, I pondered the possibility that Lola and her family would actually come and save me, and I developed a very powerful image in my mind's eye of a big black car (maybe a limo'), with tail lights glowing like cigarettes, pulling up outside directly behind me. Remembering 'Raiders', and the climactic scene, in which Indi' and Marion are tied up not far from where the Nazis are opening the Ark, I felt that I must not turn my head, because the sight of the demons that would appear would be too terrible to behold and live. (My thinking was clearly muddled or in a state of flux since, on reflection, it is clearly irrational to equate looking at Lola's family's car with seeing demons if Lola's family had come to save me.)

However, it seemed to me just possible that, if I were to move slowly enough from my seat and pull a contorted facial expression at Dave Jones, I might reduce him to a gibbering idiot and so make good my escape. (I was assuming that Angela was my ally and so wouldn't try to stop me leaving.) I think that I also felt a certain sense of shame about the way that events had turned; ie, I'd thought I'd saved mankind, but now here I was, completely involved with my own salvation. I wondered what would become of Angela. – It was now or never, and I inched my way incrementally up and out of my chair. Was I going to make it? I think that I'd got as far as having risen fully to my feet when Dave Jones laid a hand on my shoulder, and inside I knew that I'd soon be saying hello to hell.

The Total Obliteration Of Hell

A puzzling interview

I was subsequently shown into a room where I was seen by a doctor. The situation seemed laughable to me because I thought that, in my then current state, or rather, the state in which I believed myself to be, I was probably invisible to him. (It is clear that I didn't really think this through, because I didn't consider that I might be invisible to anyone else; ie, I didn't question the fact that I'd been recognized in casualty as someone waiting to see a doctor, and that therefore I must have been visible to at least somebody employed by the hospital. Perhaps I felt that I was specifically invisible to the doctor because he represented the full weight of the established medical profession, and so was blind to the psychic aspects of life and death?) However, although I was in part more than a little amused by the possible perplexity of the doctor (and the poor man certainly did look bewildered to me), I was also concerned by what I considered much more disturbing questions concerning the possible fate of my physical being. I don't believe that the thought of seeing a corpse that was supposed to be me bothered me greatly, and I was intrigued by the idea of witnessing my own funeral. But I was not happy with the possibility that, were I not 'irrevocably expired', my body might be damaged by attempts to find signs of life, and then destroyed when there appeared to be none. And I was also concerned that 'I' might feel physical pain as I was mucked about with, even though I was 'not strictly embodied'. And of course, were cremation to occur,

I wouldn't be able to return to my physical shell. I'm not sure whether I felt the full irony of the possibility that a perfectly healthy body might be destroyed for no better reason than that it was temporarily unoccupied!

The Total Obliteration Of Hell

The 'Ship of Fools'

I'm not sure how I was transported to hell, but I arrived in a good humour. 'Hell', or the 'Ship of Fools', as I very soon decided to call it; (a) because the layout seemed very much like that of the cross channel ferry, and (b), because everyone seemed like a lost soul; revealed itself as not unlike a rather shambolic pyjama party, and one of my first thoughts was to find the booze. Needless to say, my attempts at obtaining liquor proved fruitless, but there were plenty of distractions, chief amongst which was the discovery of Lola's 'alter ego'; - short, squat, and with sad, taunting eyes.

I knew at once that she was 'Delores' (Lola is the pet name for Delores, the latter meaning pain or sorrow) and, as I looked at her, 'brilliant rays like lasers' shot from her eyes towards mine, and from mine to her: - a genuine hallucination? Was this then to be my fate, in consequence of my 'star-crossed' love for the sweet and fair Lola Jimenez – to be doomed to spend the rest of eternity locked together with this 'lamentable impostor', who was effectively Lola, and who therefore still attracted me with a power too great to fight off, but who was yet very far short of the proud but happy girl who so loved life?

As I have indicated, there were plenty of other distractions. One such was the disturbing behaviour of someone called John Partridge, who was either having a fit or being sick. I thought that, in fact, he was Jim (James Stephenson from the field course), though goodness knows why, since the resemblance was hardly striking. And an inanely grinning negress also caught my attention. I christened her 'the wise virgin'; I was certain that she was a 'version' of Valerie, also from the college.

I'm not sure what time of day it had been when I'd arrived on the 'Ship of Fools', but I daresay I'd assumed that it would be permanent night-time there: - my first memories are that it was dark. I've no idea how long I'd been there when I decided, or was encouraged, to go and lie down. Whatever, I was not at all peaceful. For one thing, I couldn't shut out brilliant beams of light when I closed my eyes, and I was also not content to be resting alone. (I had decided that, whatever the disadvantages of being in hell and chained to Delores, at least I had sex to look forward to, added to which I felt incredibly tense and agitated, and it seemed to me that the soothing touch of a mature, experienced woman was the only possible remedy.) In fact, 'Delores' did 'take pity' on me, and, even though it was not in the manner that I'd envisaged, I was too distraught to argue the toss, and compliantly swallowed the evil looking green lozenge which she assured me would help me to sleep.

The Total Obliteration Of Hell

In which I go in search of Willow Walk

Strange to say, a brilliantly sunny morning followed night. I don't remember awakening; I seem to recollect dressing. I know that I was impatient to have breakfast and 'get the hell' out of hospital. (I must now have realized that this was where I was.) I was told that I'd have to see a Dr. Dhugiralah (spelling probably incorrect), and the thought of this 'interview' gave me 'the willies'. Investigating 'Lincoln Ward', where I was incarcerated, I discovered a sign; 'Fire Exit', and for some reason supposed that this meant that in order to pass this way it was necessary to use a firearm to shoot off the lock. Having no gun, I resorted to my 'special powers' and, with a hefty shove, 'forced' my way through the unlocked doors. I don't believe that I was followed (assuming that my premature departure was observed) – being the new kid on the block, I had not yet developed a reputation as an escape artist.

Outside in the chilly air, I was further convinced that something had befallen the world I used to know, and anxiously looked for landmarks to guide me as far as the entrance. Arriving at a gate with which I was not familiar, I suspected that the local geography had somehow altered, and hesitated, panicking slightly as I wondered if Willow Walk still in fact existed and, if it did, whether I was up to the challenge of locating it.

Somehow I attained the 'Ridgeway'; that grand old road, and my wilting confidence revived slightly, although I was still somewhat uncertain that the turning to the right into 'Upland's Park Road' would have been untampered with. It hadn't been affected. I believe that it was on this occasion, although it may have been during one of my later 'breakouts', that I noticed a turning that had 'appeared overnight', and which bore the to my mind sinister title of 'Vulcan Gate': - I kept straight on. I joined the footpath I had used many times as a child, and so arrived in what was now the road of the moment in my book; 'World's End Lane'. Near the end of the footpath, I became aware of a figure walking a dog some distance away, and on the opposite side of the small stream that borders the path, and I anxiously wondered whether this being was friendly or posed a threat, and tried to walk in what I considered to be an appropriately neutral manner. World's End Lane was home to my friends the Callfs', and I may have been tempted to knock at their door (see later), but home was beckoning strongly, and besides, I didn't know whom I could trust, so it seemed sensible not to complicate matters.

The Total Obliteration Of Hell

The universe runs amok

I don't remember my homecoming on this occasion, but I think that it was on this particular day that my confusion peaked for an awful few moments; perhaps the least savoury of all my experiences of instability. I was back in our dining room, and the television was on, and my father, who was in a compassionate frame, was also present. I was highly agitated physically, and was quite torn between running into dad's arms and seeking solace by 'touching' the T.V. And I remember distinctly that I was quite certain that the meaning of everything that I'd previously considered worthwhile in the universe; love, beauty, reason and so on, had somehow been distorted; ie, that 'God' had lost control of 'His' creation, and that everything good and bad was completely mixed up. It was not that I feared that evil had triumphed (even that wouldn't have been quite as awful); nothing and no one had triumphed; good and evil were equally hopeless; everything and everyone would from now on live in torment from the frustration of never being able to find rest. And of course, there was no solution in death; after all, 'I was dead', and I was still around!

I believe that later that day I was returned to hospital. Whether it was the evening of the same day, or that of the following, or at least two days later I cannot remember for certain, but it was certainly not long afterwards that I made my way home a second time, and, on this occasion I clearly recall that I had a strong temptation to ring the Callfs' doorbell on reaching World's End Lane: - there was 'magic' in the air, and I thought it quite likely that Freda (my mother's friend, and mother herself to my friends Robert, Richard and Catherine) would cordially invite me in for a drink to celebrate the 'end of the world', which I envisaged they'd be watching on television. However, once again the urge to get home was stronger.

The Total Obliteration Of Hell

Time is in reverse

My mother was not pleased to see me. She was sitting in the dining room. I think that her bad leg was resting on a stool. She looked very young. I was particularly aware of the older items of furniture in the room, and had a strong sense of time having flown into reverse, feeling that maybe it was 1960 once again, or perhaps even the 40's. I was very enthusiastic, and tried to convey this to my mother, but she seemed unshakeable in her judgement (which she did not hide) that I shouldn't have come home, and that I couldn't stay. When I realized that pleading with her further was unlikely to pay dividends, I turned to my father, who seemed clearly sympathetic. I cannot remember if I stayed at home that night, but I believe I may have done, upon the condition that I agreed to be returned to Chase Farm the following morning.

In which I fail to reach Madrid

I am not sure that it was the next day (though if it wasn't it was not long afterwards) that I made another futile attempt to get to Madrid. However, as to whether it was my intention to visit Lola when I set out this time I'm not sure since, when I hailed the black cab that happened to be passing our house at just the 'right' moment, my intended destination was my friend Simon's ex girlfriend Siggi's.

I don't know if I was anxious about the possible reaction of the taxi driver when he should discover that I couldn't pay him, but I think I was aware that I had no cash. Upon revealing my lack of funds to him on reaching Muswell Hill (about four miles from home), he was certainly not best pleased. However, for whatever reason, he did not try to detain me.

Siggi being out, I followed my nose, for want of a better description, in what I hoped was the direction of Islington: - it was now my plan to call on my buddy Phill'. I can't remember if I found his road, but if I did, he was out. Continuing my travels, I had a drink in a pub that was bought for me by 'the boyfriend'? of a girl called Jane, with whom (Jane) I discussed the 'state of the universe'; ate a meal in a 'Golden Egg' restaurant (leaving without paying of course), and wandered around inside 'Sadler's Wells Theatre': - goodness knows what I had in mind. I also chatted to a couple of bus drivers. I believe that I asked them the number of the service I should catch for Victoria; I was aiming to board the 'Supabus' to Madrid from Victoria Coach Station.

Frank Hayward

I turn myself in

I'm not exactly sure why, but I eventually grew tired of wandering about, and at length, 'gave myself up' to the police; simply announcing that I was lost. When asked to empty my pockets, I 'humorously' enquired as to whether the young policeman who had made the request was gay. Having been relieved of my worldly goods, I was invited to make the acquaintance of my own personal cell, complete with toilet and a mattress to lie down on. And, after having given up shouting for a cigarette, this is what I did; ie, lie down. The next thing that I can remember is my father being admitted to the cell. During the drive home (dad took me straight to Willow Walk), we happened to pass my friend Phill' in his car. I believe that we exchanged greetings. I don't believe that he realized at this stage that anything unusual had happened in my life, or at least, anything more unusual than usual.

The Total Obliteration Of Hell

Lincoln Ward

Back home, I was immediately struck by a most unusual phenomenon; the telephone cable stretching up the stairs and out of sight. However, I think that by this time, anything out of the ordinary seemed just par for the course. My uncle Arthur and auntie Ida were present, and the former gave me a telling off, as far as his mild manners would allow, for worrying my family: - he seemed to have little idea of the power of what I was going through. I suppose I put his remarks down to the eccentric ignorance of the English when faced with a crisis. Once again I'm not sure if I stayed the night; if so, it was the last time for weeks that I slept in my own bed.

That evening (or possibly the following morning) began one of my most intense periods of unadulterated insanity in Chase Farm. I had little idea of the passage of time, and much of the early spring of '85 is lost to me in terms of what I did on certain days, and whether in fact I was even conscious much, at least during the first week or so. I can only suppose that I was heavily sedated at first, or at least, once it had become apparent to the staff that my restlessness and agitation were rendering me rather hard to handle. For these reasons, I cannot (once again) list the procession of my experiences in any strict time sequence, and besides, one day was in many ways just like every other. However, many impressions remain vivid in my memory, some involving people, and some concerning incidents that seemed of great importance at the time. I shall begin to enumerate these by speaking about what I remember of the remainder of my spell on Lincoln Ward.

I have a distinct recollection that the first room that I occupied; possibly for the duration of my short time on Lincoln, was numbered 6, and that I associated this with the cult television show 'The Prisoner'. (The number 6 was in fact assigned to his person: - same difference.) Anyway, I supposed that I'd been given the 'toughest assignment in the hospital' – to escape from room 6. My strongest memory of this room is of an attempt that I made to read whilst sitting in bed. I don't especially remember Angela visiting me on Lincoln Ward (I believe that she did at least once), but at some stage she brought me in a book. I cannot remember the title, but I recall thinking on turning to the first page and glancing at what was written, that it was intended to enlighten me to the extent that I would find an inner peace. I don't think that I ever got past page one. I remember that it said something about fishing and a river (it certainly sounded idyllic), and I visualized the stream each time I stood in a state of tension in front of the toilet in order to help my urine to flow.

During the first days of my captivity, when the notion of being physically in a place called hell was still strong, and perhaps before I'd got friendly with anyone, the T.V. screen exerted a powerful attraction, especially the images and music accompanying the credits to 'Emmerdale Farm'. To me, the countryside depicted was really the 'Elysian

The Total Obliteration Of Hell

Fields', and I willed myself to be drawn, quite literally, through the screen into this 'wonderland', in which I envisaged having a small allotment where Lola would work by my side. I would stealthily approach the telly, pressing my fingers against the screen in an 'E.T. style touch', and feel the magical crackle of the static. Needless to say, my behaviour annoyed some people, but I was more or less oblivious. Another strong impression concerned the showing of the film 'The Eiger Sanction', starring Clint Eastwood. As the film commenced, 'he' looked haggard and uneasy, and then 'he' was shot, which was not how I remembered it, and which inclined me to the view that a worldwide madness was affecting the plots of previously 'fixed' films. (In fact, the actor seen at the beginning of this movie is not Clint, but does bear a passing resemblance to him.) And so began my fantasy that the ageing Clint would be 'reincarnated' inside my relatively young (twenty five year-old) body.

At the far end of the ward, and partially cordoned off from the T.V. room area, stood a ping-pong table, and a young man, flamboyantly attired in dressing gown and slippers, and who I fancied was the actor Dustin Hoffman (researching a role I suppose) or his alter ego, hung about here at times smoking rolling tobacco. And there was a sharp featured woman with owl-like spectacles who just had to be John Lennon, though whether in body or spirit I'm not sure. And sometimes there was an oriental nurse close by; she was presumably Yoko. I don't think that I spoke to these characters at first, but after a day or two I had developed a nodding acquaintance with 'Dustin', or 'Gelli', as he chose to be called: - 'Lennon' had apparently 'flown the coop'.

Miguelina was a short, pretty, dark haired girl of Mediterranean origin and, from the way that she danced with her hands, I took her to be a 'version' of Madonna. (The then current Madonna single 'Material Girl' was played several times a day on the radio in the ward.) Miguelina was also keen on the music of 'Lionel Reechie' as she called him.

There was a room on the outer side of the main corridor with respect to the main lounge-cum-dining room which was lined with armchairs along the walls, and which was labelled the 'Quiet Room'; somewhat of a misnomer, since it was often the case that music could be heard, apparently emanating from the ceiling. A girl (a visitor I believe) was often to be found sitting in this room in the evenings, and sometimes, when I looked again a minute or two later, she would have disappeared without a trace, only to have reappeared when I looked again after another short interval. I decided that the girl was the singer Kate Bush, and that she could appear and vanish when she chose. Another character, who came onto the ward occasionally, reminded me facially of a guy I knew called Mervin Macintosh, although this person appeared to be at least partly female, and looked as though 'she' was in the advanced stages of pregnancy. She had a singsong, rather flat speaking voice, and in this latter characteristic it was similar to Merv's voice. I

The Total Obliteration Of Hell

was baffled; was she/he the embodiment of 'Gosnawk', the mystical little god that Merv' and my friend Simon had invented? (I believe that Lisa; her actual name, was equally curious about the strange being called Frank.) And then there was a young nurse called Sally Andrews, with bubbly hair and a bright, bubbly personality and fine figure, who I also thought was in fact someone else; a Gill I'd met two years previously. I am not sure what it was that made me so convinced of this; Sally looked younger than I remembered Gill as having done, but I believe that I explained the apparent rejuvenation by supposing that Gill had been a witch (a good witch) who could change her appearance at will, and that Sally was the form of her current manifestation. I was so taken with Sally/Gill that I dared to proposition her, much to her embarrassment, although I think that she soon forgave me on account of my condition.

I'm not at all sure for how many days I'd been on Lincoln Ward when we were all relocated to 'Sussex', but I certainly remember the occasion on account of my fear upon entering the lift to go downstairs that I'd be trapped, and possibly even crushed, by the walls closing in on me.

Introducing Sussex Ward

I have a plethora of memories of the early days of my stay on Sussex Ward. One of the first of these again concerns a television set. I was now extremely restless, and found sitting down for any length of time an ordeal that was quite beyond my endurance. An elderly middle-aged man, who seemed to me to be a dead ringer for the politician Keith Joseph, and who was wearing a wine red sweater, forced me to sit down and face the screen. As to whether he was staff or a megalomaniac patient I'm not sure to this day. There was some sort of black and white film being shown, and I was captivated by the sight of the young Ingrid Bergman, who appeared to be pleading with someone. To my way of thinking, she was pleading for my soul, she being in heaven and having somehow been made aware of my predicament. I was beginning to get quite involved in the proceedings when I was summoned to the corridor; my friend Charles had come to visit me. It was a bit of an anticlimax, especially since he bore me nothing but a sheepish grin.

As I have already intimated, much of my time was spent asleep. I didn't rise or go to bed at set hours (or at least not as far as I could judge), and was quite disorientated, perhaps because of this, with regard to time. On one occasion when I left my dormitory at some stage during the day, I was particularly aware of what I regarded as the latent bewilderment of the young student nurses, who

The Total Obliteration Of Hell

seemed to be hanging around without a clue as to what was going on. One such; a lightly coloured girl; Cecile R. Moore according to her name badge, stared at me, rather boldly I felt, and I think that I asked her something: - she seemed entirely ignorant of the chaos that I discerned. My general feeling about the situation of Chase Farm at this time, both in terms of its location and its function, was that it was one of a few outposts where life was carrying on (after a fashion) following some sort of worldwide catastrophe, which had struck, or been initiated, on the night that I'd returned to England on the ferry. And for some reason, I had the notion that famous faces from the worlds of sport and entertainment would somehow get word of our existence and would arrive on the ward to provide aid.

During my waking hours, I spent a large proportion of my time on the move, walking along the corridor, which formed a horseshoe shape, and completing the circle via the day room. This, and smoking the cigarettes that the vampire-like Lavinia 'magicked' from the sleeves of her dressing gown, kept me as calm as I was capable of being. Hours would pass in this way, the radio playing songs whose words seemed peculiarly pertinent to my situation; 'Dancing in the Dark'; 'I Can't Fight this Feeling Anymore'; 'Everybody Wants to Rule the World', and another dozen or so, time and time again. Very often, the music would rouse me into an emotional euphoria in which I was quite resolutely determined that I would break the 'spell' which had made things the way they now were, and I often lowered my head and shoulders 'a la Jimmy Connors'; my 'Wimbledon' hero, announcing grandly and fervently that there would be 'no losers in my game!'

The Total Obliteration Of Hell

J dormitory

Lola was very much on my mind, and woe betide anyone who dared stain her good name. (I was restrained and given an injection at least once because of my angry reaction to someone's comments about her.) One day, on pausing briefly in front of the T.V. in the day room, I was sure that her street in Madrid was being shown on a map, and another time I was certain that she'd jumped off a bridge and had died. This led me to the notion that, sooner or later, my precious girlfriend would be 're-embodied' on the ward in one of the female dormitories. Naturally I was eager to discover her there. Accordingly, whenever the thought occurred to me, I would deviate from my course and march into 'J' dormitory (J standing for Lola's surname, Jimenez, or so I thought) and over to the bed on the right by the window: - I've no idea why I chose this bed. Sometimes there would be nobody there, but there'd be some chocolate, and I'd regard it as a gift to keep my hopes up. On other occasions a plump, ugly, and thoroughly dejected girl would be lying in bed, which would be somewhat of a disappointment, although even then I had to make sure that it was not Lola's face that was hiding beneath the covers, in addition to which it also entered my mind that perhaps 'Susan' would turn into my beautiful princess were I to kiss her gently. Needless to say, Susan was not too keen on me for the duration of our mutual existence on Sussex Ward. However, I was not altogether without friends.

Frank Hayward

'The Weetabix'

Kevin had introduced himself early on during my stay in Chase Farm. In fact, I believe that on the day of my admission he'd tried to make me welcome, but that I'd told him he was a fool: - he never let me forget this slight. I daresay that I first became interested in Kev' because he had a guitar stashed beneath his bed, and I was keen to relieve the tedium of my day by strumming a few chords. Kevin however was far from eager that I should 'work out' on his precious instrument, and it seemed that the only way that I could get hold of it was to sneakily slide it out from beneath him whilst he was resting. Invariably he would come to and tell me to f--- off, endeavouring as he did so to grab my arm. A similar scenario was enacted whenever I tried to gain access to his copy of 'Restaurant at the End of the Universe'; Douglas Adams' sci-fi sequel to the much acclaimed 'Hitchhiker's Guide to the Galaxy'.

I'm not quite sure what it was that finally dissolved this state of tension between us (maybe we exchanged cigarettes), but one evening we made an excursion to Lincoln Ward which, as I have intimated, was now upstairs from us and, during a conversation that we had in the corridor and 'Quiet Room', it dawned on me that I'd found a kindred spirit. From that moment on, Kev' and myself became a united front in dealing with whatever hardships, imagined or actual, we encountered. Along with Gelli, we adopted the collective name

The Total Obliteration Of Hell

'The Weetabix', based on the banal T.V. adverts for this cereal, and together we would 'haunt' the upstairs corridors at night, running breathlessly arm in arm and collapsing into laughter, with no more sense between us than a gang of delinquent thirteen-year-olds.

Frank Hayward

Bath time

Kevin and 'The Weetabix' aside, I was often far from content with life on the ward. One of my greatest fears, after experiencing it for the first time, was bath time. Patrick; a softly spoken and rather melancholy Irish nurse, supervised what was, as far as I remember, my first bath since my admission to the Psychiatric Unit. I daresay that, at the outset, I wasn't altogether happy about undressing in front of a male nurse. But this was nothing compared with the way I felt when he poured a sachet of orange liquid into the bath whilst running the water: - I supposed that this was blood, and that I was to become a human sacrifice! And even when nothing sinister did in fact occur whilst I was bathing, I still felt that Patrick was toying with the idea of doing away with me, and that the orange liquid, if not actually blood, nevertheless symbolized it. Likewise, whenever he gave me a shave, I couldn't help thinking that maybe he was contemplating cutting my throat.

The Total Obliteration Of Hell

Facing my father

I believe that I phoned my mother at least once during the early days on Sussex, and that I was adamant that I couldn't face my father visiting me, and requested that he not do so. (Whether this was because I still thought that dad was 'the Devil' I'm not quite sure.) I don't remember if, on his first visit, I tried to send him away, or attempted to hide somewhere, but it wasn't long before I lost my aversion to his coming to see me, even if I was a little frustrated that, each time he came, it was without the bottle of wine that I'd asked him to bring from my bedroom. In my restless condition, I was not content to sit with dad in the quiet room on Sussex Ward (and perhaps not even capable of doing so), and kept walking out and along the corridor and back again. And in this state, I was full of admiration for his ability to sit still, and for his calm demeanour, and I wondered whether in fact it wasn't I who was the 'wicked sinner' rather than he, and 'confessed' to him that I 'realized' that it was possible that God was punishing me for the style of life I had adopted, and in particular for having collected pornographic magazines. I believe that dad suggested that I might be correct in thinking this.

Another of my less savoury recollections of the early days concerns an occasion on which, perhaps because of the drugs I was on, Lavinia (the woman who 'magicked' cigarettes), and my father, appeared green in hue to my vision. I was very unsettled (not specifically because of this I don't think), and was terrified that I wouldn't be able to stop myself from smashing my head against some glass just to get all my agitation out of my system. Fortunately, I managed to drag myself back into the dormitory and to lie down and sleep it off, pondering before I slept on whether to change my name.

The Total Obliteration Of Hell

Freaked out by the T.V

As I have previously intimated, television programmes seemed to have changed immeasurably from what I'd been accustomed to before I went to Holland, and the more I saw, the more I began to regard these changes as indicative of an evil influence at work. One night in particular stands out in my mind. The Michael Winner/Charles Bronson vehicle 'Deathwish' was being shown, and it definitely seemed to have been modified; in fact, I had the uncanny notion that I was seeing, quite literally, through the eyes of 'Paul Kursey' (the character played by Bronson). Once again, it appeared that the format wasn't fixed as it used to be: - the implications were alarming. Bearing these perceptions in mind, perhaps it is not altogether surprising that I took it upon myself to push the television set onto the floor on at least one occasion: - I don't believe that the staff understood that I was 'doing everyone a favour' by nullifying the medium's 'subversive influence'!

Joey

Joey was a trainee psychologist from Florida, whose primary (and perhaps only) thrill in life, judging by what he said, was having (and contemplating engaging in) mind blowing sex. From the moment that I first noticed his presence, seated ominously in the day room in his overcoat; his spectacles serving only to emphasize his macho cool, I was obsessed by the thought that he was Lola's boyfriend (I'd met said individual in Spain, and so was in a position to appreciate a certain resemblance), which straightaway caused me to regard him as a threat. And the fact that when I mentioned Lola to him he was adamant that I should forget about her (obviously he didn't in fact know her) served only to confirm my suspicions.

One of my first excursions out of doors after my prolonged spell of confinement on the ward was when Joey took me to the hospital shop. I cannot remember precisely what was going through my mind, but I was unquestionably apprehensive, and had little faith in his motives, especially when he appeared to be trying to encourage me to steal some sweets. - I think that the fact that Kevin and Gelli seemed to rub along with Joey alright melted my reserve somewhat and, during the weeks and months that followed, we had our share of laughs around the table tennis table.

The Total Obliteration Of Hell

Boys will be boys

I'm not sure at what stage Kevin, Gelli and myself were moved into the same dormitory, but I do recall that we had some fun together. One of my latest tricks was to 'fall' very slowly out of bed, placing a hand on the floor to support me as I 'fell': - I would then pull myself back up into it again. This exercise was designed to help me to get ready to go to sleep: - I was still very restless. And Gelli derived great satisfaction from jumping on Kevin and myself and mercilessly tickling us. Opposite our three beds against the further wall, Winston Brown; an extremely paranoid coloured man in his mid thirties, would lie for hours covered by his bed sheets, occasionally summoning up enough courage to show his face and lament the supposed facts that MI5 were after him and that his girlfriend was going to shoot him. And then there was Deepak, of Asian blood of some description, who would draw back the curtains that he chose to pull around his bed and announce, with manic delight, that he was going to make a movie called 'The Fastest Gun!' I found this hysterically funny, particularly I think because he spoke so quickly. – I believe that by this stage of my 'career' as mental patient, 'Diane Chandler' had appeared on the scene.

Diane Chandler

Diane was forty two years old and, as I told her, looked like a cross between Robert Plant and Chris Evert. (I'm not sure if she was flattered.) She had a spot in the corridor near the entrance to the ward beside the table tennis table, where she would sit serenely in her pink night gown, drawing on a cigarette from her seemingly inexhaustible supply. I daresay that much of the time she probably felt like death warmed up, but she always had a kind word for me, and we became very attached; certainly on my side, although I daresay that it must have occasionally crossed her mind that I was a 'cupboard lover' as I smoked her umpteenth cigarette or sat on her bed and devoured all her chocolates. Sometimes we would play table tennis, and her 'Chris Evert side' always assured me of a good game. I was Jimmy Connors of course.

The Total Obliteration Of Hell

The Spring Dance

I believe that the Psychiatric Unit's 'Spring Dance' was held sometime during March: - I still had little idea as to such things as dates, or even what month it was. The dance was held in the Day Hospital dining room. I'm not sure whether I'd been to the Day Hospital before, but if I had, I'd certainly not been to a disco there, and the convivial atmosphere (I believe there were decorations) seemed tropically exotic after the stark environment of the ward. I don't remember a great deal about the evening; I know that I was in quite a euphoric state, and eagerly 'got drunk' on the non-alcoholic punch, and that my father and Sally Andrews were present; the latter looking her radiant best. And I also recall lying down on the floor at one stage; an action that I suspect was inspired by someone blacking out. I don't know if it was because of this that I was escorted back to the ward by a suitably robust nurse/s, but either way, my taste of the 'good life' was, on this occasion, tragically short, and I ended up being sedated by way of a needle in my rump. (It may have been that this was the evening on which I climbed over a long black car that was parked just outside the entrance of the Psychiatric Unit from bonnet to boot: - if so, maybe this was the reason for my sedation?)

Frank Hayward

'Frankie Goes to Hollywood'

The evening that the Oscar ceremony was to be shown on television I had decided that I might be due for some sort of award. And I got it into my head that I would be summoned upstairs to the top floor of the Psychiatric Unit to appear on television. And the arrival on the ward of an attractive blonde dressed in red seemed to me to be the cue that I'd been waiting for. I'm not quite sure what this award was to have been for, but it had seemed to me that for some time, the mega pop/rock band 'Frankie Goes to Hollywood' had been riding on the success of my name, and that it was time for me to be recognized; in Hollywood. I suppose that it is needless to add that the 'woman in red' did not invite me to appear on T.V. and, by bedtime, I expect I was told to get into my pyjamas (as per usual) and to take my medication and retire to bed; in fact, I don't believe that I was even allowed to stay up and watch the ceremony on T.V. Perhaps it is not really very surprising, bearing in mind what I said earlier.

The Total Obliteration Of Hell

Coffee time in the Day Hospital

Aside from the Spring Dance, my earliest 'encounters' with the Day Hospital took place when I was allowed to start taking my morning coffee there; probably initially accompanied by a nurse. As to the precise stage of my treatment at which this took place I am not certain. I do know that it was a welcome change after the weeks? of my relative confinement. It was here in the dining room that I became familiar (by sight) with many colourful characters; many more than I can immediately bring to mind. To simplify matters, I will restrict myself to descriptions of those most readily accessible to my memory.

As I grew accustomed to the daily comings and goings, I became aware of the regular arrival of a band of chunky, elderly ladies, whose members sported white permed hair (some with a blue rinse), and whose robust, waddling gait engendered the impression that each was considerably encumbered by her handbag. Furthermore, since each woman was built like a carthorse, it seemed logical to conclude that these accessories must have been made of lead, hence my name for this group; 'the heavyweights'. Gladys was perhaps the leader of the heavyweights (or heavy mob), both in terms of bulk and by way of her vociferous speaking voice. In appearance (she was bespectacled), I can best describe her as a spot on, living 'Giles cartoon granny'. However, even Gladys in all her glory was rapidly eclipsed by another woman, also of mature years, who made the rest of the brigade (to which it is highly questionable that she genuinely belonged since her hair was iron grey) look like a bunch of demure maidens. Elsie; the name of this venerable larger than life creature, once accustomed to my appearance, would make a beeline for me and plant a swift, leathery kiss on my lips with a ground shaking intensity that had me worried for fear of concussion!

Scattered around the dining room were small round tables and chairs, and it seemed to me that those people seated round the tables having their coffees were in fact conducting seances. I considered some of the middle-aged and elderly ladies to be spiritual mediums: - I included Catherine Callf's mother Freda in this category. I also felt that the number of people seated at each particular table was highly symbolic, although I'm not sure now which specific numbers I considered to be the most magical or spiritually significant.

The Total Obliteration Of Hell

O.T

The Day Hospital was not of course designed solely for providing morning coffee and meals, and eventually I was assigned an occupational therapist and introduced to the O.T. department. – As had been the case with certain patients and members of ward staff that I'd met at Chase Farm, so too did Sandra, my O.T., remind me of someone I had known before.

If I recollect accurately, I found my first days of occupational therapy a rather humiliating experience, for here was a girl barely my age, quite unselfconsciously (she was not in the least bit patronizing) involving me in the kinds of simple activities and games I thought I'd seen the last of on leaving infants school. Nevertheless, however laughable it seemed to me in my continuing euphoria, I may have felt it represented progress.

No upper age limit

At the time at which I was a patient on Sussex Ward there was no upper age limit, and, as it happened, an elderly contingent was strongly in evidence. There was in particular a 'hard core' of old/ancient women of very limited mobility. It was not long before I had got to know their names, and I would go round to each of them in turn, speaking enthusiastically and projecting 'positive vibes'. (I believe that this was my way of paying lip service to my imagined faith healing abilities.) One of these unfortunates, whose name was Mary Rushton, appealed to me enormously as she lay on her beanbag next to the television; her round face and glasses giving her the appearance of an owlet. She loved being kissed, but such an undertaking was not without risk, for sometimes she would bite. Her main occupation, apart from waving her amazingly pliable limbs about, was to repeatedly utter certain phrases, of which I remember 'foonee finger'; at which she would display a bent digit; 'I'm gooing round', and 'where's Alice?' I thought that she was referring to Lewis Carroll's 'Alice', but in fact Alice was her sister. I believe that it was Mary Rushton in particular who inclined me to the view that perhaps I was in 'purgatory' rather than hell, for the poor woman was everlastingly trying to grasp for something beyond her reach. Whilst Mary may have appealed to me in particular, each member of this 'posse' of geriatrics stood out by virtue of his/her individual behaviour and appearance. Lillian was the archetypal witch, with her lank white hair, pointed nose, and thin rasping voice which poured forth vitriol. In between her utterances, she would spit with unerring accuracy. Doris was skeletally thin, and had eyes that seemed to be lost inside her head. She would pipe mournfully like a curlew for her morning weetabix. And then there was Russell, the token man, and a loveable rogue not easy to love, who must have been one of the most frustrated men on earth, with so much to express and yet such a stunted ability to speak clearly: - as if having one leg amputated to the knee was not enough.

Frank Hayward

Lola on my mind

Throughout the period of my relative incarceration, Lola continued to be very much on my mind and, in addition to my fantastic notion that she would be 'reborn' in hospital, I also often wondered whether in fact she had arrived of her own free will and was following me around, and that the only reason I couldn't see her was because she was always behind me. (I daresay that such an impression could be classed as symptomatic of paranoia, but that would I think be to misconstrue my tender feelings about her supposed presence; ie, I had no desire that she should stop following me: - I didn't feel persecuted by 'her'.) In accordance with this equally bizarre idea, I was sure that I could see her standing behind me when, in the toilet, I looked at the shiny bolts on the water closet and saw her distorted reflection. 'She' was wearing a multi-coloured sweater, and her hair was as I remembered it, hanging down over her shoulders. But the more closely I looked at the bolts, the more 'Lola' would recede behind me. A third theory that I considered (which could be said to have sprung from the second) was that Lola was now a part of me and no longer existed as a separate entity, either with or without a body. In case this was so, I adopted what I considered to be Lola-like expressions and mannerisms to 'make her feel at home'.

The Total Obliteration Of Hell

John Partridge

My obsession with Lola got me into trouble again when I took it upon myself to declare my love for her in writing in the front of John Partridge's Bible. I was lucky not to get punched by the irate owner; fortunately, staff were on hand. Much as I had no wish to be him, I was decidedly envious of John Partridge in that he seemed to have carved out a niche for himself on the ward; a position which afforded him certain freedoms seemingly outside my grasp: - he could for instance get dressed and leave the building whenever he wished (or apparently so), and he never seemed to be without a supply of temptingly long cigarettes. Needless to say, he regarded me as being beneath his contempt, and I guess that it was appropriate since he was, both physically and mentally, way out of my league, besides which, he knew the ropes. I associated a book that I often saw in his dormitory; 'The Way', with what I believed to be his mission in life; ie, 'walking the way'. (I rather doubt that it was in fact a Taoist book.) However, much as I admired Partridge for beating the system, I was not unaware of certain weaknesses in his makeup, perhaps the most significant of which was that he seemed quite incapable of keeping his supposed brilliance to himself. This tendency to show off did not apply solely to his cerebral powers, but also to what he clearly regarded as significant physical prowess; namely, standing on his head in the middle of the day room.

Frank Hayward

In which I go for a walk with 'Isadora Duncan'

As the weeks passed and I made no further endeavours to escape, so I graduated in my 'career' as patient to the extent that I was allowed, with permission, to walk on occasion in the hospital grounds. My principal port of call was the hospital shop, for here, when I had received some 'pocket money', I could indulge my passion for sweets and chocolates. But my most memorable excursion did not involve the shop. I had recently cottoned onto, or she to me, an elderly middle-aged woman who, whilst not good looking, was certainly of striking appearance, and whose name; Isadora, was also suggestive of all things esoteric.

My excursion round the grounds and through the general part of the hospital with Isadora was a revelation to me. For one thing, Dora took a great interest in the stones and litter beside the path, collecting certain items (I can't remember what specifically) that she described as 'diamonds'. I was fascinated, not having witnessed such behaviour before, and I believe I joined in, although I don't remember for sure if I kept any souvenirs. I do have a vague memory of a chewing gum wrapper which had printed on it something to the effect that I was lucky. Dora disappeared briefly whilst we were investigating the main building, and I was a little nervous in case she didn't return and I'd be 'lost', but she wasn't gone long, besides which I became engrossed by the behaviour of some small children who were playing with a bar football table. Having

The Total Obliteration Of Hell

by this time been confined so long to the company of adults (and youths), I'd forgotten that 'smaller versions' existed, and these children were to me both strange and quite miraculous: - it seemed almost inconceivable that such small beings could function so intelligently. – At length, we returned to the ward just in time for lunch, and presented the staff in the office with a brick that we'd collected on our travels: - I don't think I quite understood why Isadora had picked it up, but it all seemed to fit somehow.

Frank Hayward

My impressions of the ward staff

In addition to a plethora of student nurses, including the delectable Sally Andrews, and 'virginal' Ruth (more about whom later), Sussex Ward was manned by a number of permanent members of staff and, although I did not at the time regard them either as friends or even professionals genuinely concerned with my welfare, my retrospective impressions of their characters are not I think entirely lacking in affection. This is perhaps particularly so in the case of a short, curly-haired Mauritian named Dave, who was assigned the task of watching over me during the time at which it was felt likely that I would make another bid for freedom. Naturally enough, the dutiful attentions of this viceless little man were not in the least welcome as far as I was concerned; in fact, I think that it was precisely this diligence, coupled with a 'terminal', mild mannered pleasantness, that bugged me so much.

Every time that I thrust open the double doors at the entrance to the ward and strode defiantly off down the corridor that led to the outside he would be on to me, pleading with me to return and tugging at the sleeves of my jacket. In my frustration with him, I rather impolitely named him 'the toad in the hole', on account of his liquid brown eyes and, in my 'mobile' state of mind, I sometimes actually believed that he really was a toad in human shape; perhaps one that I'd kept and handled against its will? On the rare occasions when I had time for

The Total Obliteration Of Hell

Dave we played table tennis, and he developed the habit of asking me whether I would like to give him 'another roasting' whenever he had a mind to play. Ultimately, Dave told me that he was returning to Mauritius to run his family's sweet shop, and I can honestly say that, by this time, I was genuinely sorry to see him go. But not every member of the ward staff was as humble and unfailingly kind as Dave.

Jonathon was the hard man of the crew, and, perhaps partly because of his menacing appearance (though it probably had more to do with the fact that he held quite a senior position), was the first to appear if anyone 'threw a wobbly'. Sharply featured and curtly spoken (though never gratuitously rude), he appeared to take his work very seriously, and had no time for pleasantries. Sometimes I thought that it was in fact he who was 'the Devil', and secretly I called him Jack. – Amongst the women there was of course 'Delores', whose name was in fact Nelda; Li, a little Chinese nurse whose temperament was rather similar to that of Jonathon; bold and brassy Mel Carpenter, who looked like a gypsy with her raven hair, and Malandra, with her cunning 'Mona Lisa' smile.

Ruth

In addition to Sally Andrews, who left after six weeks or so for University College Hospital, Ruth (I don't remember her surname) holds a special place in my memory amongst those student nurses who were 'attendant upon me' during my spell in Chase Farm in the spring of '85. From my first sight of her, I was quite convinced that she was in fact a girl I'd had a crush on at Middlesex Poly'. However, if she was, or had been, she clearly didn't remember it. I decided without further ado that, this being the case, she could be none other than 'Ruth' from the Old Testament. And, gazing into her blue eyes, I was equally sure that 'Ruth' stood for 'truth', since one so innocent seemed incapable of telling a falsehood. In appearance, this maiden (and maiden she surely was, since it was impossible to believe that she had ever even been kissed) was not unlike the physical type preferred by Renoir, and here she was in her childish red shoes, with nothing better to do than sit about with me, raising her feet so as not to obstruct the domestic who was washing the floor. I was not in love with her, oh no, but I don't deny that I marvelled that she had 'fallen into my lap', especially when she offered to get me stamps for my letters to Lola. However, this blissful period was short-lived, since (and I'm not sure how the subject came up) Ruth betrayed her 'goody two shoes' image by telling me that she thought that Lola was 'horrible', and, after this slight to my true love, I was never quite as comfortable with her again.

The Total Obliteration Of Hell

A significant night?

It was, I believe that I'm correct in saying, well into my stay in hospital that I spent much of one night pacing about my bedroom and up over the bed; pausing to examine my naked physical form in a mirror; convinced that I was going to metamorphose into a 'new' person. However, I do not recall any disappointment the following morning when I was unable to discern any visible change. (I wonder whether the events of that night, and this reaction of acceptance of my 'fixed self' the next day, marked a turning point in my condition; ie, the point beyond which I no longer needed to regard myself as akin to a Messiah? But I am speaking retrospectively; I was not aware at the time of any sudden revelation to this effect.)

Frank Hayward

Home for Easter

Easter was fast approaching, and it was at length agreed that I might have some home leave. I was 'over the moon', having often felt that I was doomed to live out the rest of my days on the ward, or that whatever had happened to me had involved irreversible damage to my brain and nervous system in general: - it now appeared just possible that fate was going to give me another stab at a meaningful life. However, I was not without certain reservations, especially regarding my ability (or rather the lack of) to stay in one place and settle my attention on a particular subject or task. But I was unquestionably elated by the prospect of seeing my precious bedroom once more, and being able to get outside and smell the spring air.

If my memory serves me correctly, the first occasion upon which I was officially allowed home was a Saturday afternoon. I believe that my father picked me up in the car: - I'm not sure if I stayed the night. My abiding memory of this visit is rather unpleasant, since I was afflicted by a raging sore throat for about an hour, and could do no more than lie on the sofa in our lounge and wonder if this was part of some divine punishment. I think that I also managed to have a 'heart to heart' with my father, and I believe that it was on this occasion that he gently sermonized to me. From what I remember, this was in response to a rather confessional mood on my part, along the lines that I might be sensible

The Total Obliteration Of Hell

to forget my ambition to live with Lola and start a lizard farm on the outskirts of Madrid.

On one of my first official trips home, I managed to type at least one letter. This boosted my confidence somewhat, although I was rather concerned whilst engaged in this activity by the noises of construction emanating from our kitchen. I must have been more than a little paranoid, for I feared that my father was making a wooden cross to nail me to! I didn't consider this to be an evil action on his part, in fact, I wondered whether it might not be an inevitable consequence of my past sins; ie, he wanted to purify me.

Another activity in which I engaged shortly after being allowed home was gardening. My father supervised this. He seemed very patient but, although I wanted very much to get into the swing of the task, I found the intricacy of the work quite beyond me and soon gave up. Dad was very attentive to me during my first home visits; playing the piano for me, giving me wet shaves, and just being around to lend a listening ear. He even conducted a psychological test on me based on my colour preferences. I'm not sure that he ever told me what he'd concluded from the results, but I believe that he said that my liking for grey indicated depressive tendencies.

My mother still being laid up in bed with a thrombosis and sciatica, I saw rather less of her than of my father, but I remember chatting to her on one occasion as she sat up in bed. I think that I'd brought her a cup of tea, and perhaps this pleased her; at all events, she seemed a lot less like Hitler, and even appeared to have a vague inkling of what I was trying to get at when I suggested that the world had recently experienced a kind of madness: - I think that I mentioned how strange television programmes were these days and that she readily agreed.

My earliest official trips home to Willow Walk were quite sacred as far as I was concerned; I wanted to soak up everything that I remembered as having been pure and good; everything that I could trust and didn't need to slough off as worthless or dangerous. As a consequence, I hardly touched a cigarette during my weekends (this abstinence later went by the board), and revelled in the privacy of my room and good company of my family. If I had a real problem, it was that I was spoilt for choice in terms of things to do, and rather lacking in the conviction to choose and, having chosen, carry anything through without being tempted to try something else instead. So I flitted from my typewriter to my lizards to studying the 'Radio Times': - even this appeared to have changed dramatically. Everything was glorious, but I felt a bit foolish in the face of it all, and found to my disappointment that, at first, one night at home was all I actually wanted to spend, and that, perverse though it may sound, I soon began to crave the 'treadmill' of the ward and incessant smoking.

The Total Obliteration Of Hell

PART 2: 1986-87

The 'relighting of the boiler powering the central heating of my heart' was inexplicably, and inextricably, linked to the waxing of the autumn of 1986. I had been uncomfortably and uniformly numb for many months and, perhaps because of this, was quick to sense the slight surge occasioned by this 'reignition'. I was not to know that this desperately craved for relief from the apparently inescapable depression that it had been 'my lot' to endure since the summer of the previous year was not only a sign that my 'emotional swing' had begun to move again, but also a warning that I should not abuse the return of the precious gift of the ability to appreciate existence by becoming greedy and 'swinging right over the top of the swing'.

Frank Hayward

In which I find some relief

The first indication I can now recall of the commencement of a shift in the balance of my mood relates to my powers of verbal expression; in short, I began to converse without effort to my nurse in the Day Hospital: - I had completely lost this facility in the aftermath of my madness of the previous year. Whether or not it was wishful thinking I don't know, but I was sure that Nicki (the nurse) picked up on this 'exhumation' of my personality, and that she was glad of it. I, in my turn, was grateful for her apparent appreciation. With the return of a significantly greater verbal (and consequently social) ability, so I became aware that I was not quite as uncomfortable in myself in terms of how I felt physically-cum-psychologically about the 'burden' of consciousness, particularly in relation to my perception of duration. However, as to whether I felt better because I could express myself more easily, or vice versa as I suspect, it wasn't long before the 'river', for so long dry, began to flow once more.

I believe that it was on a Sunday afternoon, although I daresay it's academic, when I really 'pushed the boat out' and became ever so slightly enthusiastic about water-colour painting again. It is true that I'd found a certain amount of solace through sketching in pencil on occasion during the long depression, but this was somehow different; I felt an opening up of possibility and, perhaps most noticeably of all, was no longer smoking '19 to the dozen'.

I was still attending the Day Hospital for occupational therapy during the early part of the autumn of 1986. I cannot recall the full extent of my programme of activities, but I was certainly involved (as a patient) in what was referred to as the 'Young Persons Group'; a fairly informal social club for the under 30's, and, as what had been for so long no more than barren existence became a meaningful life again, so I actually began to look forward to the cinema trips, walks etc in which we indulged as 'Young Persons'. However, as my confidence grew, so did I become rather opinionated about what we did. I suppose I felt that I was now in a position to be a helper rather than a patient. A particular instance sticks in my mind in this regard; it has to do with an occasion on which we went swimming at a local pool.

Frank 'knows best'

Mary Quigley was a rather peachy looking, and very young, O.T. who, it seemed to me, found it difficult on occasion to be assertive. On this particular afternoon, she had taken it upon herself (I daresay quite properly) to help my friend Michael with his swimming. I was exploring the water in strange new ways, and having a good time, and it occurred to me to suggest to Mary that it might be better were Michael to be left to explore technique on his own. Poor Mary seemed rather put out by what she clearly felt to be interference on my part. – Another example of my growing ego was when I was loudly critical when we went to see the movie 'Top Gun' at a local cinema.

The Total Obliteration Of Hell

In which I gain a job and a chameleon

I believe that it was very close to the end of October of 1986 when I finished at the Day Hospital to take up part-time employment on a government training scheme based at 'Trent Park'. Roughly speaking, the purpose of this particular project was to survey the flora and fauna of local parks, sports grounds etc. When I first got the job, I had to attend a short induction at 'Enfield Civic Centre'; basically no more than filling in a long official form. I believe that I was by this time sufficiently sold on my supposed personal importance that I felt distinctly impatient and critical of the other people sitting around the table when they took a lot longer than I to fill out the form. When I began this job, which paid £64 per week for twenty hours work (to me quite a princely return), things certainly seemed to be looking up; - the work was a source of some satisfaction since it related to wildlife conservation, and the 'heavy' wage packet made ample provision for the 'resurrection' of my hobby of keeping reptiles and amphibians just as my enthusiasm for this (and for my interests in general) was beginning to return apace. And of course, there was plenty of time to indulge this interest, since I was only working three days a week.

I started keeping copious notes about the lizards, toads and newts that I acquired (I had not done this for a long time), and became relatively obsessed with constructing aesthetically pleasing displays of plants, rocks etc to fill the cages that my charges occupied. Perhaps, in so far as it relates to my 'volatile' health, my most telling purchase was a large chameleon. I think that I am correct in saying that I bought this in early November, though I daresay that the exact date is purely academic. During my return from the shop with my 'strange cargo', I went to see a social worker in the hospital. The chameleon stayed out of sight in a polythene bag under my jumper. Perhaps on reflection, even this 'risque' behaviour on my part might be regarded as the action of someone slightly unbalanced? But maybe I'm just being 'wise after the event', and besides, I don't suppose that the risk of discovery was that great, and the lizard had ample air.

However, as the weeks passed subsequently to my acquisition of this apparently venerable, and 'stereotypically prehistoric' beast, I began to feel slightly unsettled by the 'looks it gave me' as I stared at its rotating eyes, and formed the conclusion that I in my turn was causing it upset. My solution was perhaps quite rational; I bought another bushy plant to give it more privacy. But I couldn't keep from my conscious mind the disquiet I felt about the chameleon's eye contact with me, and, in what I now consider to have been a paranoid condition, imagined that it was 'giving me the evil eye'! This unpleasant notion was not a constant preoccupation however, and on balance, I was quite proud of the chameleon, and spent time photographing and sketching it, and observing its ponderous, but almost unceasing, daytime activities, and frequent changes of colour and

The Total Obliteration Of Hell

pattern. Sadly, it did not thrive for long, dying after a mere six weeks or so on 31st December. However, although it could be argued that this was, at least in part, a reflection of my deteriorating ability to look after it as a result of my own by that time 'sad' state of health, I am reluctant to form such a conclusion, since the maintenance of chameleons in captivity is not without its problems, and I'd been remarkably unsuccessful with the two I'd had previously, long before my mental health was in question.

Frank Hayward

'Swings and roundabouts'

According to my mother, November '86 was about the time that she really began to feel human again (not her words) after a period of dark depression, prefaced in September '85 by an overdose of sleeping pills; a desperate response to worries about my father's physical health and my failure to get over my breakdown. Dad had subsequently taken early retirement; ie, whilst mum was in hospital in the autumn of '85; partly to keep things ticking over at home, and partly because of his own failing health. Just before Christmas '85, he went into hospital himself. I later learned that he had been operated on for cancer of the prostate. – By the summer of '86, he appeared to have made a good recovery, but then came pains in his arms and shoulders.

He spoke casually (to reassure us?) of a relatively innocuous condition called 'polymyalgia'. But whatever he may have suspected or feared, the fact was that his mobility was becoming increasingly restricted; eg, it became a supreme effort for him to climb our stairs. Under these circumstances, taking a stroll was quite out of the question for dad, and I took to going for walks in the park with my mother: - she claims not to remember these. For my purpose, one particular walk is worthy of mention since, whilst on it, I revealed myself as quite a troubled man; weeping; shouting; refusing to adopt mum's route round the lake, and abandoning her on a low wall, calling her a 'cold

The Total Obliteration Of Hell

woman', because I suppose she had not comforted me to my satisfaction.

Frank Hayward

All downhill 'til Christmas

I continued to be employed at Trent Park as autumn shaded into winter. My friend Robert Callf had now also joined the scheme, primarily as a bird recorder, he having some amateur expertise in this field. For a while, although it cannot have been more than a few weeks, I was content with the position, and I was particularly proud of the fact that since I'd started there, I'd reduced my consumption of cigarettes whilst at work to nil, having my first of the day when I got home at 5 p.m.

However, as my sense of self control, and corresponding feeling of security grew as I took a greater command of my smoking habit, so just as surely did minor differences of opinion with my work colleagues become a source of anxiety and, as in February '85, my social instincts proceeded to desert me although, on this occasion, paranoia was perhaps more pronounced, especially in the portakabin that constituted the workplace. But the paranoid feelings were not very concrete either; ie, I wasn't convinced that I couldn't trust anyone, I just wasn't sure whether I could or not, and if I could then who. But perhaps I'm rather jumping ahead, since I don't believe that the paranoia really sprouted until after the Christmas holidays, since I was still sufficiently socially intact that I was able to enjoy and be a part of our Christmas lunchtime drink (with my fellow workers), and to have a discussion afterwards with Robert about ethology.

The Total Obliteration Of Hell

But it was not only in the work environment and with my mother that I became easily upset.

For some reason, I took an immediate and intense dislike to the curate of our local church; ie, that attended by my parents, and was decidedly cool to him when he passed me on the street on one occasion. His reaction was to put it to me that perhaps I had forgotten him; I found this suggestion inexplicably insulting. Upon returning home, I made a great 'song and dance' to my parents about this incident. My father was sympathetic over the extent of my distress, but I suspect that in fact he was considerably more concerned for the balance of my mind. On another occasion, my uncle and aunt paid a call to our house, and Tom; my mother's brother-in-law, enquired about my job. His manner had always grated on me and now, in desperation and furious defiance, I responded by lying down on the floor, presumably to the consternation of my relatives. I had to contend with uncle Tom again on Christmas Day, but somehow managed to rise to the occasion and do no more than mutter derisory comments under my breath. Christmas Day 1986 was particularly poignant for our family, perhaps particularly in retrospect, although even on the day, the extent of my father's physical incapacitation was unquestionably of concern to all present. (I believe that the journey we made to south London that day was the last drive dad ever made at the wheel. My mother assures me that he also drove us home, but my memory of it is that my brother Peter did so.)

Frank Hayward

I come off medication

It is perhaps pertinent (some would say unquestionably so) to point out that I came completely off the low doses of drug medication that I'd 'officially' been taking at about the time I left the Day Hospital. This did not just represent 'deliberate forgetfulness' on my part, though I may have secretly hastened the transition. I certainly remember that I weaned myself off 'Temazepam' sleeping tablets (the 'evil looking green lozenges' mentioned in part 1), but I did confess to this action to one of my nurses and, to the best of my knowledge, this step did not meet with Day Hospital disapproval.

The Total Obliteration Of Hell

An over-impatient outpatient

To the chagrin of my ego, leaving the Day Hospital was not even a temporary 'final farewell' to Chase Farm, for I was made an outpatient. This meant of course that I still had to see a psychiatrist for a check up every so often. In fact, as it turned out, the only appointment that I was given prior to my readmission in January '87 was somewhat of a nightmare to me and, on reflection, I can well appreciate the doctor's (apparent) scepticism as to the chances of my maintaining a degree of equilibrium as far as my state of mind was concerned. I have suggested that I was not truly paranoid until after Christmas, and my outpatient's appointment was before then, and I was unquestionably suspicious of the doctor and anxious about the appointment. However, although it might be argued that my suspicions were unjustified, and therefore clearly paranoid, it seems to me that a certain amount of concern over meeting a relatively unknown quantity with some authority to reinstate me in the Day Hospital, and possibly the ward, and the power to put me back on medication, would be quite natural; ie, I am suggesting that a degree of worry that I might never be free of the hospital's clutches would have been quite normal even in an individual quite well balanced psychologically. But that is not to say that the almost obsessional fear that I exhibited prior to this appointment with a man who (to my mind at the time) was aggressive and power crazed, could be considered indicative of someone of entirely sound mind. (I should explain that I had met this doctor briefly prior to the appointment; he was introduced to me whilst I was having lunch in the Day Hospital.) The extent of my emotional disruption was even more greatly emphasized by my anger and frustration when the original date of the appointment was changed because the doctor in question was off sick; ie, I'd psyched myself up for the occasion, and now I was going to have to go through the whole process of being anxious and trying my best to calm down all over again. In the event, my worry over the possibility that I might be put back on medication etc remained no more than that; the doctor simply saying that, were I to feel subsequently that my condition was deteriorating I should let it be known so that appropriate action could be taken. I'm sure in fact that I heard him say 'when this should happen' rather than 'if', but perhaps I was so 'freaked out' by this 'forcefully charming' African that I heard 'when' because I assumed that he had it in for me. (It could of course be that he did indeed consciously choose to say when rather than if because he was sure that I was already going off the rails, and wanted to warn me without actually saying to my face that I was going downhill fast.)

To cite one further example of the 'borderline paranoia' that I was exhibiting towards the end of 1986, I would mention my anger at my father upon discovering that he had made a tape recording of an argument (or should I say a shouting match) that I'd had with my mother a day or so before. I don't know if it was the fact that he had concealed this action from me (I only discovered it by accident) that infuriated me, or more that I remembered that I'd made some offhand remarks of a decidedly racist nature about the doctor, and was concerned lest the tape be handed over to the hospital authorities, but perhaps this latter possibility concerned me more than the concealment?

I have used the term 'borderline paranoia' because, much as my reaction might be posited as evidence of paranoia, once again it seems to me that it was not an entirely irrational one. However, as 1986 gave way to January '87, there is now no doubt in my mind that I was lurching ever more frequently beyond the boundaries of my everyday world of reality.

Frank Hayward

Some beliefs that I held in January 1987

There now follow some examples of the more dramatic, or perhaps melodramatic, notions that underpinned my strange new world.

(1) I thought that 'Frank Hayward' died during this month, and that 'I' now existed in order to rectify the misconceptions that I felt existed concerning 'his' 'former life'. I regarded 'him' as having been a visionary, who had not received the appreciation and respect that 'I' deemed had been due to him for having been such a 'wise and loving' person.

(2) (In rather the same vein.) I thought that 'I' was now no longer human, but a step beyond on the evolutionary ladder, to which I gave the name 'self frigging hermaphrodite'!

(3) I thought that my mother was evil.

(4) I believed that my reptiles and amphibians could thrive on air and water alone, and that it was best to leave the tops of their cages open, so that they would have 'more freedom'.

(5) I thought that I was number 1 in the hit parade, even though 'Top of the Pops' wouldn't admit to it.

(6) I thought that the world had lost its ability to love, but that I still knew how, and that, eventually, when people became sufficiently desperate to find the love they'd lost, I'd be there to show the way.

The Total Obliteration Of Hell

I will touch on some of these points in more detail as the tale of the events of early 1987 unfolds.

In which I experience 'bodily emptiness' for the first time.

I arrived back home at Willow Walk late on in the afternoon of January 1st 1987, having spent the night of New Year's Eve at Phill' Franklin and his girlfriend's flat in Islington. I believe that there was no one at home when I arrived - my father had been admitted to the general side of Chase Farm; I'm not sure where my mother and brothers were: - I don't believe that I was disturbed by their absence – I may have expected it. I had enjoyed the New Year celebrations (if I remember correctly I'd indulged in some of my 'notorious' dancing), and was I think in a tranquil frame of mind. I don't remember anything about the rest of that day apart from the fact that I watched a bit of 'Star Wars' on the T.V. for the umpteenth time.

I don't remember for certain the date on which my work at Trent Park recommenced after the Christmas break (possibly January 9th); at all events, I believe that I was happy enough to return, even though, in the event, one of the first tasks that I was required to undertake saw me getting rather flustered. I cannot recall the precise nature of this mission, but it involved going to the civic centre in Enfield Town and taking something with me; some form or other. I was a bit on the late side on the morning in question and I couldn't find the form, and was hunting high and low for it amongst the mass of paraphernalia in my bedroom and getting myself in a 'tizz'. I'm not sure if I found what I was looking for, but I do remember jogging up Slade's

The Total Obliteration Of Hell

Hill in the snow, and of being conscious of the thought that the motorists in the traffic queue stretching down the hill could all see me and that I was very self-conscious about it: - decidedly paranoid? Having left the civic centre, I reflected on the behaviour of a young female receptionist whom I'd addressed: - she had seemed to have been half asleep. I can't remember now for sure, but I believe that I thought a thought along the lines of there being a dull state of awareness amongst those who worked at the civic centre, and that this thought led me to suspect that this was a syndrome affecting office workers in general. I may have explained the lethargy in terms of the heating in offices being turned up particularly high, and I believe that I considered the possibility of a connection between this 'winter dormancy' and the long winter in 'Narnia' during the reign of the evil witch. As I undertook the journey to Trent Park on foot, I felt decidedly pious to be bothering to show up in such severe weather, and I had a wonderful daydream about phoning Lola and inviting her over for a cosy lunch-time drink in a dimly lit pub. (I'm not sure why I remember this so well; perhaps it related somehow to one of her letters, or to a telephone conversation we'd had?)

I'm not entirely sure that I bothered to go all the way to the prefab that day. However, increasingly disturbing perceptions and fantastic ideas notwithstanding, I continued to attend my place of work, and to function more or less as I gathered was expected of me, right up until (and including) the day of my 27th birthday: - January 15th 1987.

Frank Hayward

The snow on the ground and chill in the air were extremely invigorating, and offset to a certain extent the disquiet in my mind over such things as my boss's unshaven, red eyed appearance (which struck me as distinctly demonic), and the whispering of two of the girls on an afternoon on which I was alone with them in the hut: - I suspected that they were plotting to torture and murder me!

We didn't drive around the district much during what was my final week at Trent Park, but several of us walked about in the snow to a certain extent and, on one such occasion, I had the sublime feeling that the substance of my body had entirely melted away and that I was no more than a spirit with the external appearance of a physical being. The feeling of having no body mass (I didn't feel light, just void) was wonderfully liberating in itself, but perhaps equally satisfying to me was the accompanying notion that death need no longer concern me. Curiously enough, on another occasion (possibly even on the same walk) I felt distinctly uneasy, sensing that my life was in danger as long as I continued to walk alone in the snow. Whilst the feeling of physical emptiness was most pronounced on this one occasion, I was also frequently aware of feeling that my weight was changing instantaneously as I moved about. This was curious, but not unpleasant. Perhaps more disturbing was the apparent pitching of the floor of the prefab. I had felt this rocking once before, after my return from the Netherlands, and it hadn't augured well then. I was also (now) aware of a

The Total Obliteration Of Hell

slight ache at the base of my spine. It seemed to me that this sensation was affected by the position in which I stood or sat in relation to my colleagues. On this note, I especially remember an occasion when everyone else in the hut was sitting on high stools and facing away from me towards the long work top running from end to end of one side of the prefab, whilst I was seated on a low chair on the other side of the building facing their backs. I felt certain that, were I to sit on another high stool with the rest of them, it would alleviate my suffering. (Regrettably, there were no more high stools.)

Frank Hayward

In which I experience 'death'

Trent Park contained a college (now university) campus, and part of my work on the wildlife project involved using the college library. However, one of my final actions involving this repository was certainly not work related, since it consisted of writing a note in one of the subject catalogues about the absence of a heading for 'love'. I cannot remember the wording I used.

During the final day or two of my employment, my thought processes were exceedingly sluggish. I'm not sure if I was especially distracted from what I was doing by paranoid suspicions, or whether it was simply that, whilst remaining focussed on what I thought was the task in hand, my mind simply wanted to stay where it was rather than 'dredge up' the next thought. I was also very short on sleep.

For a week or so prior to being readmitted to hospital, I cannot remember sleeping at all. I was excited by 'strange phenomena', and by what I had started to feel (as I had in '85) was a special, crucial role for me in the workings of the universe. With regard to the 'strange phenomena', one example is the 'fuzzy air' that I perceived upon removing my glasses. (On reflection, I suppose that this could be simply explained in terms of a heightened awareness of what things look like to a myopic person not wearing spectacles; ie, as opposed to a genuine hallucination.)

The Total Obliteration Of Hell

As I stated earlier in my list of six fundamentally flawed beliefs that I espoused at this time, I thought that I died during January '87, and this belief (an appreciation of which is central to the vaguest understanding of the extent of the 'displacement' of my former sense of reality by another) is intimately connected to my sensory perceptions of the aforementioned strange phenomena.

Prior to 'dying', I had decided to make a break with my family; not by physically leaving, but by living alone in my part of the house: - I don't think I'd worked it out beyond that. I suppose that my increasing ineptitude at social interaction, even with members of my own family (who I probably felt were seriously inadequate intellectually to be my companions, and who seemed quite indifferent to my fate); paranoid mistrust of the basic integrity and worthwhileness of almost every living being, and an arguably almost inevitable, inwardly-turning obsession with my supposed uniqueness as a sort of prophet or voice in the wilderness, combined to create a situation in which all that was required was a tiny spark to 'inflame the rotten edifice of the life that I'd been living'. (That is rather melodramatic but, however it might be expressed, there was definitely a shock wave coming, and the impact was going to be profound.) (In case it appears that I was aware of this at the time, I should stress that I was much too involved with the tide of emotion and sensation to reflect, even assuming that I'd been capable of doing so; no, I may have realized that it was a momentous point in my personal history, but history has to be enacted, and act I did.) – Perhaps it's time for me to stop presenting my interpretation of this time of instability as fact, and simply relate, as best I can, the events of the evening on which I experienced 'death'.

Prior to turning in for the night, I observed that my mother and younger brother Tim were in the dining room. I think that they were sitting in the dark; I particularly remember the glow of the electric fire. I don't know if I bid them goodnight but, if I remember rightly, I sensed that they were a twosome; two family members joined by a bond of mutual understanding, and that I was an intruder. As I went upstairs, feeling like a spoilt thirteen-year-old, and momentarily aghast as I suddenly thought that perhaps I was mentally retarded but too stupid to have ever realized it, I developed a yen for a roll-up and began, on reaching my bedroom, to search for tobacco, becoming increasingly desperate when no half finished pouch was to be found. I'm not sure if I was in my pyjamas, and didn't like the thought of redressing and braving the outside world to go to the off license, or if I was certain that it would be closed, or if I was prepared to go but couldn't scrape enough money together; whatever, I endeavoured to enlist the aid of my brother Peter. I found him singularly unhelpful, perhaps because he couldn't understand why I wouldn't settle for an ordinary cigarette. I can't remember whether I also asked my mother to help me out, but if I did, she declined. As she mounted the stairs and turned right to her landing, I turned left to mine, yelling at the top of my voice that she was an a—hole; so loudly that it seemed to me that I could expect

The Total Obliteration Of Hell

thereafter to be celebrated in the neighbourhood for having stood up to the 'evil Esme Hayward'. And as soon as I entered the sanctuary of my bedroom, it dawned on me that something momentous had happened; I'd at long last shattered completely the bond that had, physically and emotionally, like it or not, tied me to my mother's 'apron strings'. I don't know that I saw it in quite those terms at the time, but there was no question in my mind that I had freed myself from bondage to a monster! However, along with the relief, there was apprehension related to (a), the psychological insecurity of my 'new condition of freedom', and (b), what was to happen next. I also felt a morbid sort of pity for the 'old dragon': - would my having 'ripped our mother/son tie asunder' be a mortal blow to her, and would I find her cold and dead in her bed the following morning? (I doubt that I gave the possibility that my mother's interpretation of the evening's 'events' might be at variance with mine a second thought.)

As to whether the 'empty body' sensation was prompted on this occasion by the 'stunning realization' that I was having I know not, but, sure enough, once again I felt physically void. As I stated earlier, when I had had this feeling the first time (in the snow in Trent Park), I had felt a tremendous sense of peace. This time however, I was slightly unnerved by the sensation, wondering how I could move to my bed and lie down when my arms and legs were 'no more than shapes'. (I may also have considered the possibility that going to bed was no longer appropriate, being as I now considered myself bereft of physical substance.) At all events, I remained awake for hours, contemplating the possibilities, and possible consequences, of having 'ceased to be a flesh and blood being'. And, just as had been the case in 1985, so I wondered whether I was no longer visible to the living, and, if so, whether I could carry on a sort of existence indefinitely in the house as a form of ghost. I also conjured up scenarios in which my family would enter my room looking for me, and would either find a corpse and have it taken away, or else, if I was not to be seen, conclude that I had at last decided to leave them in peace, and that the best response was simply to leave 'me' or my 'ghost' be and continue their own lives.

The Total Obliteration Of Hell

The last strange days of my freedom

As to whether the night I have just described was in fact that immediately preceding my readmission to the Psychiatric Unit I cannot clearly remember, but I suspect that it was not, since my friend Keith Broadbent visited me shortly before my readmission; probably on the night of January 15th (I was returned to hospital on the morning of the 16th), and I do not associate the night of the above events with his visit.

About a week prior to January 16th, I appear to have stopped making notes about my reptiles and amphibians. (The last entry that I subsequently found was for January 5th.) As I mentioned earlier in connection with my work at Trent Park, my thought processes had become very slowed down, and perhaps this accounts, in part at least, for this cessation in writing. But perhaps it had more to do with my rather dreamy and disoriented frame of mind when I was in a room on my own. I was not entirely unaware of my trance-like state, since part of me was still trying to make the effort to engage in the activities I was accustomed to enjoying, and I distinctly recall striving to follow things through in my mind. So lost was I, that I was quite consciously worried that, once alone in a room, I would never find my way out again. My ultimate escape at this time was to run a piping hot bath and, as the vapours rose, surrender to a 'mist of enchantment'. (I may have related bathing at this time to the song 'The Lamia', from the album 'The Lamb Lies Down

On Broadway' by 'Genesis': - I had been playing this L.P, and it seemed to echo the strangeness of my experiences.)

On January 15th 1987, the date of my 27th birthday, I trudged home up Snake's Lane in the snow from the prefab in Trent Park for what was to be the last time (in relation to this particular job). I was on my own, and accepted a lift from a well-to-do man with glasses driving a posh car, whom I regarded with disdain; not visibly I hope, as far as Oakwood Station. As I walked along Prince George Avenue, I was struck by the beauty of the afternoon, but there was something more; my visual reality was transformed for several minutes whilst everything; people, cars, road and trees 'became' a fantastic, Disney-style, Technicolor cartoon. Were you to ask me now to put a finger on what exactly it was that was different about the view from the way it usually appeared, I would have to say that it was the way that I was regarding things that was different rather than what I was regarding.

I seem to remember once again arriving home to an empty house, but that there was some black forest gateau in the fridge, as if by way of consolation. I think that I went and lay down on my bed, feeling like an actor after having looked in my wardrobe and possibly having changed my clothes. I do not recall sitting down to dinner.

On one of my last evenings of freedom we experienced a power cut and, when candles were lit, I was reminded of a scene in the shock horror

The Total Obliteration Of Hell

film 'Carrie'. I was intensely concerned that my brother Tim would be blinded; either by looking too directly at the candles, or by the sodium lights when they came back on: - he was positioned so as to be able to see this happen.

Another of my most vivid recollections of my last nights at home was my waking dream. In this 'dream', I was lying unclothed on a bed spread with a white sheet. Purple curtains surrounded the bed, perhaps four feet away from it on all sides. And, standing alongside me, were all the women/girls with whom I'd ever been infatuated, with the exceptions of Lola and one other girl, Claire, with whom I'd been particularly smitten. Although these girls were also naked, my feelings were not explicitly sexual; it was a peaceful scene, as if they were waiting in attendance on me, and I equated them with angels, bade to provide me sublime comfort by way of their grace and beauty. Largely at peace, I awaited the arrival of Lola. I sensed that she would be bashful about making an appearance. I also thought that Claire might show up, and this possibility concerned me somewhat, but I reassured myself with the thought that if she did try and enter the house it would be to no avail, and that she'd get buried in the snow. This seemed fitting since, at the time, I felt that she was a demon from hell! As the dream faded, I had still not managed to conjure Lola into appearing, but I do not recall feeling especially disheartened.

The night on which my friend Keith Broadbent came to see me, I assured him that I was dead, and gestured eagerly at the '2nd Krishnamurti Reader', which I had previously borrowed from him. I think the inference was that I'd fully digested it, and was now exhibiting behaviour that corresponded to a realization of its infinite wisdom. I'm not sure if I offered him coffee or if he was 'obliged' to ask for a drink, but some time later I was vaguely aware that my mother was boiling a kettle downstairs, and that this social task had somehow eluded me. I remember little else about the visit; maybe Keith looked slightly bemused when I suggested, as I believe I did, that I was 'Indiana Jones', but I don't think that I would now remember his 'I don't know what to make of you' expression were it not that subsequent realization that I was not okay at this time had led me to reexamine everything that had transpired. (It is of course possible that being wise after the event has encouraged me to be overzealous in interpreting past events as pointing to instability and delusion.)

The Total Obliteration Of Hell

A lamb to the slaughter

When Keith came to 'take me in' on the morning of January 16th, I do not recall feeling that it was inevitable that I would be readmitted to the Psychiatric Unit: - I may have felt that it was likely that I would be. At all events, I didn't have to be coaxed into leaving with him; I think that I sensed that it was appropriate, just as I had when Angela and Dave Jones had come to collect me almost exactly two years previously. However, although (and perhaps this was surprising) I displayed no sign of paranoia towards Keith during the car ride or when we first arrived at Chase, it didn't take long once with the doctor for me to sense that I had been betrayed.

Four of us were present in the room in which we were seen by Dr. Akootoo that morning; the doctor; a nurse who I knew well of old, and who everyone referred to as Matey (short for Maria Teresa); Keith, and myself. Outside, snow remnants streaked the ground much as had been the case when I'd tried to break away from my father in Groveland's Park two years before. – Having from the outset dismissed Dr. Akootoo as a potential ally, I paid little heed to his bold, wide eyed speech and flashing teeth, and settled my gaze on Matey for some sign of reassurance and understanding. However, I found no comfort in her expression, which I interpreted as a triumphant, 'now we've got you!' sneer. I don't know if I had assumed that Keith at least would be my advocate, but it didn't take long for me to realize that he had no intention of 'crossing swords' with the professionals; in fact, he seemed to be quite happy to go along with them. In my desperation, I expect I raised my voice, but by that time I think that I must have known that mine was a lost cause. As a final gesture of resistance I flopped onto the floor, rather in the manner I'd done when my uncle had asked about my job. – As to whether I received an injection of a powerful sedative at this point, and fell asleep, or simply blacked out I'm not sure, but I cannot remember being transferred to the ward.

The Total Obliteration Of Hell

Of women, hell and self importance

The next thing that I remember was being seated in an armchair next to a radiator beside the nurses' station on one of the wards, and being brought a plate of fish and chips. A phrase was going through my mind; 'the last great joke 'til lunchtime', and I associated it with my uncle Tom; I don't know why. I was also strongly of the opinion that I was a long term prisoner, and I felt proud of this, although I don't think that I was aware of doing so at the time.

Having eaten my 'cod', chips and peas (a repast that I remember fondly in spite of my predicament), I believe that I spent much of the afternoon in the same chair, with my left arm resting intermittently on the pale yellow painted radiator, withdrawing my hand at intervals when the heat began to cause me discomfort. Once again, I am not sure as to the precise order of events, but it may have been on this first afternoon on Suffolk Ward that I spent some time thinking about the 'Garden of Eden'. Anyway, whether or not this was the day on which I considered this subject, it certainly entered my mind at an early stage of my captivity, leading to the conclusion that women were basically untrustworthy, since Eve tempted Adam. And this made me wary of the female nurses who were, or so it seemed to me, after something special that I possessed (some sort of insight into the human condition I think) which they were willing to try and trick me into revealing, upon which they would I felt sure take credit for the discovery and pervert its meaning. (I am not sure whether I felt wary of men also; I believe that my opinion of them was not high but that I felt they were harmless, whereas I regarded women as essentially dangerous because they were out to manipulate the foolish male sex and were endowed with a powerful sense of cunning.) I also thought about my friend Kevin o' Sullivan, and wondered whether he really was James Dean as he'd suggested in '85. And I think that it was about this time that I coined the expression 'The Total Obliteration of Hell'; it seeming to me that the 'purpose of the universe' could not be fully realized as long as there was 'a hell'. (I am not sure as to whether I had a clear idea of what I meant by 'hell' at this time, but I believe I had a mental picture of the molten core of the earth.)

Another of my notions, which developed over a longer period than that about the supposed untrustworthiness of women, concerned an 'imaginary' time in the past when all animals and humans were given names (probably related to some long forgotten childhood tale). And somehow I was present in this scenario, and because of what seemed to be big-headedness on my part (I had all the answers concerning the naming of all the creatures, and wouldn't keep quiet), I was given an injection to burst the bubble of my ego, being told; by a woman?, that it would only be 'a little prick', when in fact it was aimed to eradicate me!

The Total Obliteration Of Hell

Suffolk Ward

I believe that the ward on which I was a patient at this time was 'Suffolk', as opposed to Sussex, on which I'd previously spent most of my time; ie, in 1985. I have memories of sleeping in at least three different rooms during this stay; ie, 1987, two of which were dormitories and one a single room, but as to whether I resided first in the single room and was then moved to a dormitory, or was in fact moved about in a more complicated sequence, I really cannot remember for certain. However, whilst it is once again probably beyond my powers to chart my 'progress' chronologically, I suspect that those memories that are vague and fragmentary in the sense that they seem to be separated by large black spaces of unconsciousness, pertain to events that occurred during the early stages of my time on the ward, since the vagueness and darkness suggest heavy sedation, and/or an inability to think clearly because of the intensity of my psychosis.

Frank Hayward

A guy called Lawrence

I had been aware of Lawrence previously in the Day Hospital (he had been wearing a green shirt) but, when he introduced himself as my neighbour on the ward, I'm not sure that I remembered either having seen him before or about the shirt. He had the 'side-room' next to mine a matter of days (maybe more – maybe less) after my admission on 16th January. (To be perfectly honest, I really have no idea at all whether in fact my brief acquaintance with Lawrence started in January; I had no idea of day or date at that time.) – Lawrence was very friendly (perhaps he was Liverpuddlian, although I do not recall any strong regional accent), and I think that his 'neighbourliness' and 'brotherly concern' convinced me that he was fairly stupid, and ignorant as to the extent of my 'not inconsiderable' social skills! I don't know that I was aware of thinking in these terms at the time, but I do suspect that I was frustrated by my relative inability to express myself clearly and to assert myself; ie, I believe that I had to 'suffer the fate' of hearing opinions other than my own. (I should add that, in all fairness to Lawrence, I don't remember a single word he said; neither do I recall any subjects upon which he may have touched.)

My clearest memory of this time is a mental picture of myself and a rather earnest, bossy, and cheerful young man, together and alone in a room lit by yellow light and surrounded by darkness.

The Total Obliteration Of Hell

Of lying in bed

The fact that many of my memories of what I believe was the early part of my stay in hospital in 1987 are of lying in bed and endeavouring to rest peacefully presumably relates, in part at least, to the extent to which I was sedated at this time. One such set of memories includes the delusion of thinking that, once dressed in my pyjamas, I was perfectly secure, and could not come to any harm from an external source once my feet had left the bedroom floor; as if my bed were an island surrounded by a force field. Such a belief was quite a comfort bearing in mind the paranoid fear I had of being approached.

Another component of this 'set' (although it could in some ways be regarded as belonging to another group, particularly since it involved what seemed to be a different room) was somewhat along the same lines; ie, my bed being an 'island', but was not as comforting, since it consisted of the notion that this island was a night-time prison; a momentary sensation that I felt on one occasion when the sole of my bare foot touched the floor inclining me to believe that this was strongly heated in order to ensure that I didn't get up until morning, by which time the heat would have been turned off. My thoughts along these lines mushroomed, until I supposed that what was really happening on the ward at night was a rather sinister form of behaviour modification, aimed to turn patients into 'programmed zombies'. A girl called Imelda came to mind in this regard. Imelda had until recently seemed quite fun-loving, but had become 'suddenly' withdrawn. I related this to her wearing headphones and listening to a 'Sony Walkman': - I supposed that she'd been fooled into using this, and had been hypnotized by messages on a cassette. I became convinced that the 'ringleader' of this 'behaviour modifying cult' was the chief night man Donald, whose round face led me back to my past thoughts of the 'Moonies'.

A third memory of lying in bed concerns my 'Shirley MacLaine fixation'. The memory in question is quite singular, and rather 'off the wall' when presented out of a broader context. (I will refer more extensively to the details of my interest in Shirley later, but for now perhaps the following explanation will serve to lead into my description of my crazy and terrifying notion.)

I had become obsessed by the idea that Shirley (MacLaine); the American actress, was determined to meet me. I suppose that I felt that my belief that she had heard of the 'Frank creature' through (quite literally through) the T.V. screen, had drawn her to seek out this 'little nobody'. I sometimes felt that Shirley knew how desperately I wanted to be with Lola, and that she was prepared to help me out with my problem. I also sometimes felt that I was better suited to being with Shirley than with Lola, and often fantasized about the 'rich tapestry' of the world of Shirley MacLaine, and how much meaning she had given to my life notwithstanding the fact that we had never actually met. And from this

The Total Obliteration Of Hell

sense of purpose that I had found in the life of this 'icon' (initially through her representation of characters on screen, but more extensively as a result of reading her autobiographies), I developed the idea that Shirley and myself were like two interlocking pieces, and that the force of the attraction between us, were we to be in close proximity, would be so great as to have disastrous (physical) consequences. In short, I feared that Shirley, having finally realized the meaning of life, the universe and everything by having tapped into me and combined the power of my mind with that of her own, would come rushing into my room like an express train, and that the last thing I'd see this side of oblivion would be her face, alarmed and horrified as she realized too late what was about to happen. – And so I would lie in bed quaking, imagining my head shattering like an exploding planet, and contemplating the awful thought that I would inevitably not only be destroyed myself, but would also be unavoidably responsible for the annihilation of the world's 'most inspiring individual'! (As to whether I got as far as actually counting down the minutes and seconds until impact I cannot remember.)

Frank Hayward

My father is alarmed

As I have mentioned already, my father was admitted to hospital at the end of December 1986; ie, Chase Farm. One afternoon in what must have been early January (it must have been early in the month because I still had my freedom), my brother Peter, my mother and myself were informed, whilst visiting dad on 'Napier Ward', that he had cancer. (He may in fact have told us himself.) As to whether we were supposed to infer that the condition was so serious as to be unlikely to respond to treatment I am not sure, but I believe that although my reaction was not one of shock, I did consider that this might very well be the beginning of the end of his life, or at least, that it was a significant turning point. I visited dad on a number of occasions, both before and after I was admitted to the Psychiatric Unit. It is probably true to say with the benefit of hindsight that most of these visits, particularly those which took place after my admission (and my father knew that I was in hospital again), were not the happiest of occasions from his perspective, even leaving aside his condition: - my mother has since told me how alarmed he was by my behaviour. I had attributed his wide-eyed stare to his having gone blind! As I look back on it now, I can well understand his concern since, on at least one occasion, I tactlessly burst in on him, pulling back his curtains whilst he was sitting on some sort of portable commode and, and this is perhaps more telling, failing to have the social grace to retreat in embarrassment Whether through plain fear at the

The Total Obliteration Of Hell

thought of the possible consequences of my apparent instability I don't know, but father didn't really lose his temper with me during any of these short visits and, in my restless and easily distracted state, I was left with a lasting impression of a humble, stoical individual who was 'good at suffering'. When dad was later taken home to Willow Walk for a week or two (prior to the final weeks of his life, which were spent in a hospice), I would often, whilst sitting captive in the single room to which I was often confined on account of a tendency to escape, think of him back at home 'suffering for love', and wonder if he was undergoing his 'time in purgatory' whilst still mortal. – I would like to add that, on at least one of my visits to Napier Ward the atmosphere was less strained, and on one such occasion dad became quite animated, in a gentle way, talking about bats: - apparently they fascinated him.

Frank Hayward

Sam

A nurse called Sam looms large in my memories of Suffolk Ward. Perhaps this can in part be attributed to the fact that he was (and to the best of my knowledge still is) built like a 'brick outhouse'! However, it probably has more to do with what was unquestionably a rather deluded view that I developed of him as an 'archetypal black villain'. In truth, poor Sam never harmed me as I constantly morbidly fantasized he would, and if he ever took the mickey out of me, and I'm not sure that he ever even did that, it was hardly to be held against him considering my wicked racial slurs and general belligerence. But, whether or not I could be considered mad to do so, I lived in almost permanent terror of Sam right from my first contact with him, when he used to sit outside the door of my side-room. He would be speaking in hushed bass tones to someone, and then something would stimulate him to raise the pitch of his voice and it would sweep up to a whooping peak of mirth or outrage before plummeting again to the dark depths one would expect from someone of his size. But to me, whether he was shrieking or speaking in a low pitch he was equally sinister, and I imagined that he was a black 'King Herod', out to murder me whilst I slept, this according with my idea that I was somehow involved in an important way with the 'Second Coming of Christ'. But my greatest fear involving Sam was at bath times; Sam supervised my bathing. I have already mentioned my misinterpretation of the behaviour of a nurse who

The Total Obliteration Of Hell

was involved in my taking a bath in 1985, particularly in relation to the orange liquid used (this was in fact a cleansing lotion), and the recollection that no harm had befallen me allayed my fears that I was to be a blood sacrifice; my main concern now was that I would be beaten up. I particularly recall my dread that my 'jailer' would smash my head against the taps. In the event of course, nothing untoward occurred, and I was relieved that Sam bade me wash my lower torso myself. However, in spite of the fact that I could find no fault with the manner in which Sam treated me on these occasions, I suspect, although I don't remember for certain, that I tended to feel after each bath that I'd had a lucky escape. It could be suggested in retrospect that perhaps Sam and Patrick were quite unaware of the extent to which I was frightened in my deluded condition by the supervised bathing procedures they employed, and maybe this is a point worth considering in future when staff are dealing with paranoid patients. (N.B. It may be that my bathing was supervised only after I had tended to overfill the bath.)

Much as my relationship with Sam involved deep mistrust, and frequently intense loathing on my side, and what must have been at times more than a little annoyance on his; as time went on, I began, even if only rarely, to see a softer side to the man I'd mercilessly showered with verbal abuse. On at least two occasions I was particularly aware of him working on some notes, and was somehow able to open my heart sufficiently to appreciate that, much as I might have maligned him, maybe he was only doing his job. On one of these occasions I had come to sit in the office, presumably because I had nothing better to do and Sam, quiet as a lamb, was attending to some official business. He was eating a sandwich and, and there was no reason for him to be so charitable, offered me a part of it.

Despite his size, and the fact that he was at least ten years older than myself, Sam could move quite swiftly, as he demonstrated more than once when he managed to grab me and drag me back inside the building when I'd tried to escape. On at least one such occasion he caught up with me just as I'd reached some steps, and had to disengage me from a metal handrail, which I'd grasped in the vain hope that he would be unable to dislodge me: - this must have been quite a comical sight! Perhaps even more amusing, though presumably Sam didn't think so at the time, was when he supposedly slipped and muddied his immaculate shirt whilst in pursuit of me. I did not see this happen myself since, as one might expect, I was too busy making a beeline for the main gate. I believe that it was Shona who told me about it afterwards.

The Total Obliteration Of Hell

Shona

As to whether it is ascribable to a mental condition not typical of her or whether it was simply in her nature, Shona was unarguably the 'wild child' of the Psychy' Unit that spring. Delicate to behold; a waif with spindly arms and legs, and a pretty, fine featured face sprinkled with freckles, Shona was nonetheless possessed of a tongue remarkably adept at verbal violence, and she frequently claimed to be a 'black witch'! I had first been made aware of her some time before this admission, when she had been hobbling around the Day Hospital with her leg in plaster, pouring forth vitriol like a cross between a 'Barbie doll' and a geriatric spinster. I'd not got too involved.

I'm not sure if Shona was already in residence on Suffolk Ward at the time of my admission in January, but either way, I do not recall being aware of her presence until some time later when, in the 'Quiet Room', I was struck by the behaviour of a young, and colourfully attired, female (who only afterwards did I recognize as the girl I'd seen before in the Day Hospital) in the act of illustrating the exposed (she was not indecent) portions of her body with a felt pen. I don't remember engaging her in conversation at this time, and neither do I recall the circumstances under which I began visiting her side room. But the nature of my attraction to this location is perhaps less unclear, and can I think be subsumed under three headings; (1) (not necessarily the most significant, though perhaps the most obvious 'pull'), she was attractive and stimulating in my eyes; (2) she had access to cigarettes, and (3) (this applied once I'd first visited her room) her colourful and varied knick-knacks were strong reminders of Lola's flat. It may be niave to suggest that Shona in any way welcomed, or grew to enjoy, my visitations, but it did provide her with plenty of opportunity to vent her spleen. Nevertheless, although quite how or why I'm not sure, some sort of fragile bond did develop over the ensuing weeks, and on one occasion, after she'd moved to another side room, she had softened sufficiently towards me to be willing to perform an 'act of homage' to the 'new Krishnamurti' (one of the vast retinue of titles by which I cared to refer to myself at this time), anointing me with some sort of lotion (possibly hair gel?), and vowing to be my 'first disciple'. As to quite what had impressed her sufficiently about me to show such (albeit momentary) devotion it now seems hard to imagine, but maybe it had something to do with my determination when it came to 'doing a runner'; ie, I was not entirely lacking in spirit myself. I suppose that, in all honesty, I regarded Shona as a titillating, loud-mouthed, self serving, overgrown teenager (she was in fact 24), who would live fast and die young and violently. I often thought of her as a tragic case of a child-woman whom no one really cared for, and who would as likely as not be 'aborted' by the night staff for being a runt who was more trouble than she was worth. But I was captivated by her fierce spirit, and was always pleased when she bounded back along the corridor after a day or weekend away, scrupulously greeting everyone in sight. My fondest memory of Shona is of her sitting on my lap in the Quiet Room wearing some most becoming spectacles, and referring to herself as my 'miniature psychoanalyst'; a title I had applied to her. On this one occasion, she seemed perfectly at home as 'Superman's girlfriend'!

Frank Hayward

Dora

It was probably whilst sitting in the armchair next to the radiator by the nurses' station as I often did, that I first became aware of a large presence frequently seated opposite. I don't think that I was wearing my glasses much at this time, for I would stare myopically at this gargantuan figure in her Latin yellow sweater and scarlet skirt, hugely curious to discern her features through what I perceived as 'fuzzy, radioactive' air. Quite when I decided for certain that this being was simply posing as a mortal woman I'm not sure, but it did not take me long to make up my mind that Dora was really a mother goddess, whose proper station in life was to gaze stonily down from a pedestal in the snow-capped cordilleras of the Andes; specifically the 'north-western part of north-western South America': - in short, an ancient stone statue somehow made mortal by world events, and shipped from the New World to offer her wisdom to help save, or at least direct, mankind.

Having adopted this somewhat imaginative idea, I soon came up with what seemed to me to follow on from this; namely, that it was my task to see that, eventually, she be returned to where she belonged, in what I stubbornly believed was called Andorra. (Months later, I was a little nonplussed when I failed to find a principality in South America of this name when studying a world atlas, especially as I'd frequently visualized a map of the Andes with 'Andorra' on it, just north of Peru. And I was also rather crestfallen when Dora insisted, once we'd assumed familiar roles, that she came from Cyprus and not South America.)

Whether or not because I regarded her as something more than an 'ordinary mortal', I invested Dora with special powers, including being able to appear and disappear at will, and having the ability to 'fix' faces by her eye contact. (In point of fact, I often felt that people were appearing and vanishing; ward staff frequently seemed to materialize out of cupboards when it was time for their shifts; ie, rather than entering the building conventionally. And, although I singled out Dora as having supreme power to modify the physical appearance of those at whom she looked, I also often thought that I was in danger of being turned to stone by eye contact with members of the night staff.)

Regarding Dora as an incarnation of a goddess, I was both in awe of her, and incalculably flattered that I could actually speak with her, and I loved to listen to her lilting voice, it seeming to me that both the tone and content of her speech were highly appropriate for a deity. However, I was sometimes a little troubled by her references to 'electrics', and I got the impression that the physical environment of the ward was bad for her health whilst in her 'mortal state'; eg, the fluorescent lights. (As a spin off from this, I began worrying about the possibility that my reptiles were suffering as a result of being kept in cages lit by 'electrics'.) My belief in Dora's supposedly phenomenal powers was also sometimes a source of disquiet, perhaps because I felt that, in her eyes, I must seem almost incomparably insignificant, and that, whilst she, by virtue of her 'true nature', was inextricably and fundamentally tied up with world history, I, notwithstanding my 'unusual intelligence', was basically of little note, and was in danger, should I not read the developing situation correctly, of being 'wiped out' for interfering with complicated global issues for the sake of my personal, petty desires! It wasn't that I sensed that Dora in any way meant me harm, but simply that, as a goddess, she would I felt quite naturally serve the common good without fear or favour, whereas I was primarily concerned with my own 'salvation'. On this note, one particular occasion stands out in my memory. I had escaped, and had made it to Willow Walk, and was in the dining room, where my father, his face like alabaster, and a confessional fear and acceptance in his eyes, was seated in a wheelchair.

I was elated, but deeply aware of the hopelessness of my trying to stay in the house for long. I was nevertheless keen to try and turn the situation around by some stroke of genius that would 'save the world' and would, by so doing, remove the need for me to return to hospital. And I had a plan. My father had, not long before, purchased a new hi-fi (it may in fact have been a leaving present from his workplace), and I was adamant that something positive could be achieved if I could only figure out how to use it to play Madonna's single 'Open Your Heart', which I had recently acquired: - to my mind a truly wondrous record. In the lyrics of this song,

The Total Obliteration Of Hell

reference is made to turning a key to open a lock and, to my (deluded) mind, Madonna, personifying woman as siren, and therefore being a source of danger through enchantment, was in fact posing a cryptic challenge to 'break her spell'. This would take place, or so I figured, if I could accomplish the seemingly impossible task of getting the record to play. (I don't know that my thinking was all that clear, but I sensed a cosmic connection between Madonna and Dora: - was the popular singer, for all her flashy, tarty image in fact, on a deeper level, the expression of Dora's will?) I was slightly desperate, for I was sure that Dora was silently 'calling my soul' back to Chase Farm, as if I were a silly child trying to assume the mantle of a superhero, and probably for the wrong motive. Dad however, for all his frailty, was my ally and, as I for once listened to him, and followed his painstaking instructions, a surge of hope welled in me and, to my amazement, the precious vinyl sprang to life, and for once I could taste a victory.

Anna

Although I do not in any way doubt that I lived the experience, it is not without a certain reluctance, based on a lack of conviction born and raised since my life reassumed a more familiar, dare I say normal, course, that I speak of how Anna 'became Lola' during the spring of 1987. What I have to say has not in fact so much to do with how it 'came about', for this was something which I neither questioned then, nor have (perhaps strangely) considered since, but simply concerns a depiction of the scene. So I will not attempt to gloss over the fact that I have no conscious recollection of first being aware of Anna, or endeavour to trace the development of my obsession with her (as 'Lola') any more than to observe that, however inappropriately in terms of age and appearance, she did fulfill the function of 'being the Lola I'd dared hope would materialize, virginal and new, in hospital'.

That Anna was indeed Lola I don't think that I consciously doubted for a number of weeks. Her relatively aged appearance in a sense fuelled my belief, since I was able to explain this as a sort of 'karmic punishment'; perhaps for her stubborn refusal to give in to me. But whatever the explanation for her appearance, I did not doubt that Dora's 'face fixing abilities', coupled with the right clothes and makeup, would effect an amazing transformation, and that the face I loved would be 'restored' without pain or trouble. Further

The Total Obliteration Of Hell

confirmation that Anna was indeed Lola was provided by a frequent visitor to the ward; a red-faced business type who seemed pained to see her, and who was I was sure my one time peer Robert Olivier, masquerading as her husband. So certain was I of the 'bitter truth'; ie, that one long past night of drunken passion at the party I'd held when Lola was 'first' in England in 1982 had somehow created the necessity for the two casual lovers to be bound together now as partners, that I confronted my 'erstwhile male friend' with what I was sure was his true identity, and flung his, or rather Robert Olivier's, old sports' jacket, which his mother had passed on to me, at the miserable couple, to show the extent of my disgust at their 'sham of a relationship'! It is perhaps fortunate for Anna's husband that I am a coward at heart, and not prone to jealous rages; in fact, bearing in mind my relative lack of inhibitions at that time, and the strength of my conviction that his wife was 'my Lola', it could be suggested that he got off pretty lightly! Anna was not quite as lucky in this respect, since I did become slightly amorous now and then when 'Bob' wasn't around, but even from her point of view I could hardly be considered much of a threat, since her stoical 'go-way' (she didn't speak much English) was quite sufficient to incline me to stop bothering her.

I think that it was when my certainty of her being Lola was beginning to crumble that I tried to discuss the matter with her. She didn't say much, but, at the time, I sensed that in a strange way she understood. (Either shortly before or shortly after this, I called Lola's number in Madrid whilst Anna was 'home for the weekend'. Lola sounded like Lola, and not like Anna, but I still wasn't sure that it wasn't Anna to whom I was speaking, on the basis that she had flown back to Spain for a day or two to temporarily readopt her 'more customary lifestyle'. I don't believe that I mentioned Anna to Lola on the phone; after all, if 'she' was fooling me, she'd hardly be likely to let on.) I clearly remember telling my consultant about the curious matter of 'Lola being Anna', and I still wonder whether, had he been more forceful, he could have shattered the illusion, or delusion.

The Total Obliteration Of Hell

Some more on Lola and saving the world

There are many other characters, both staff and patients, and visitors, who I encountered during this stay in Chase Farm, who are dear to my memory, and about whom I could happily indulge in conversation. However, for now at least, I feel that I ought to say a bit more about the view/s of the world and beyond that were circulating in my mind during my captivity. Whilst these notions cover a wide range of subjects, there are at least two things that are common to all of them; namely, (1) they all involve my being a very special individual, and (2) they all pertain to broad questions of life on earth and beyond; the hospital appearing to be very much at the centre of world politics and, more fundamentally, central to the vital consideration of the 'spiritual nature of mankind'. I have a feeling that this will not be an easy task, probably because, in the state of flux in which I was living at the time, my ideas came and went like bubbles, to be blown and then released; ie, it may be necessary to extrapolate from the fluidity of my thoughts rather than simply presenting them, in order to make any kind of sense.

Krishnamurti; a recently deceased spiritual master, once described the individual human being as a 'microcosm of the cosmos'. And perhaps it was on this basis that I once wrote in a letter to Lola that she 'was the universe'. Of course, if she, as an individual, was a fully self-contained whole, then so was I, so it is not strictly in the spirit of this idea that

I wanted Lola and myself to become a couple, whose union would unite the world. However, at the time, I was consumed by my attachment to the idea of our getting together, and I doubt that such considerations carried much weight with me, if indeed they even entered my head. No, I was carried away by a glorious vision of winning Lola being the way for the world to be as one; our union supposedly symbolizing the possibility for paradise on earth and, by so doing, effecting the coming into being of this paradise. And it seemed to me perfectly in line with this that all my favourite celebrities should help me to achieve this 'clearly desirable' end. I was especially keen that Shirley MacLaine should be involved, since she had always represented the very brightest and most loving aspects of the human condition as far as I was concerned. And Lola herself, in spite of her pride, could surely not help but fall in love with me for the sake of peace and joy on earth! But despite my enthusiasm, and refusal to entertain any thoughts that my 'vision' was no more than a deranged fantasy, even I was not oblivious to the possibility that Lola, and even ridiculously intelligent Shirley, might not see the goal ahead as I did. Still, I was prepared to be a 'voice in the wilderness', and besides, in Lola's case, my ego was so swollen that I had not the faintest doubt that the extent of my 'devotion to her' could not possibly escape her notice, and found it easy to convince myself that the power of my feelings would far outweigh her relative lack of physical attraction to me. On this note, I often sensed that I could hear the sweetest, mellowest voice on the radio, and that it was Lola telling the D.J that 'her boyfriend' was so stupid that he'd do anything for her. And her tone suggested that she was more than two thirds towards falling in love already. But there was also a slightly more 'intellectual/scientific' question frequently on my mind that seemed to me might help solve the riddle of human existence, namely, the identity of the character 'David' referred to by Shirley MacLaine in her 'Out On A Limb'.

It is possible that I was interested in this character because he might be a perfect 'soul mate' for Shirley; ie, it would provide some confirmation of the truth of the notion that some beings were created to be together: - I of course felt (or wished to believe) that Lola was for me and I for her. And it was my belief that, in the cause of the pursuit of the answer to this question, Shirley MacLaine and Clint Eastwood were often upstairs in the Psychiatric Unit at night in conference with my consultant. I would, accordingly, often take the lift to the third floor, enthralled and terrified by the thought that I might come face to face with Clint when the lift doors opened. Of course, I was secretly hoping that, whilst on the upper floor, I'd be invited to join in with this discussion that I believed was taking place. I felt a bit like Cinderella before she was invited to the ball.

Frank Hayward

'Frank the revolutionary' and 'World War Two Time'

At more or less the same time that I considered the question of the identity of 'David' to be of global importance, I was also somewhat preoccupied with the idea of leading a non violent revolution; in fact, I felt that, to a certain extent, this was what I was already doing. I regarded the magazine 'The Peoples' Friend' as being my revolutionary newspaper; I suppose that the word peoples' was suggestive to me of revolution! - I called my 'revolutionary organization' something like the 'One man revolution to save the entire world', or something equally humble! As to whether the idea of revolution was originally related to the then upcoming general election I'm not sure (I think not), but I do remember that this approaching event occasioned at least mild interest on my part.

It seemed to me that the most significant political issue in Britain, and possibly the world, had something to do with 'P.M.T.' and, for some reason, I had the peculiar idea that whoever won the election would do so because they had expressed a strong policy intention to keep the 'rate' of premenstrual tension either up or down.   When I say 'up', I'm not suggesting that I thought that a party that promised to increase pain amongst women would be likely to, or ought to, win: - I'm not sure what I thought that this rate referred to. (Presumably the idea of a rate comes from the plethora of political statistics concerning such factors as unemployment and inflation.) I think that

The Total Obliteration Of Hell

my growing feeling that my revolutionary party would be unlikely to win on June 9th 1987 was very much related to this matter of P.M.T. and to other 'womens' issues' since, in point of fact, I felt a bit of a charlatan in claiming to espouse female concerns, and I suspected that I would be recognized as such. I often felt a slight queasiness in my stomach, which I regarded as my attempt at empathy with the female condition, but it never seemed that bad. – Allied to the feeling I had that I was a fraud to claim to speak for women was another guilty feeling, relating to a conviction that the world was overpopulated, and that no more babies should be born: - I sensed that such a view could only point to the psychological profile of a mass murderer!

As the time of the election approached, I was sure that Margaret Thatcher often passed me on the top floor. 'She' looked quite different from the way she did on T.V., and seemed small fry by comparison with 'Clint' and 'Shirley'. My 'interest in politics' was not limited to contemporary peacetime Britain and the approaching general election, but related also to my conception of global warfare, which distinguished 'World War 2 Time', and the 'Third World War', which was either approaching, or had in a subtle manner already begun. 'World War 2 Time' was to me an 'atmosphere' that I sensed to be present on the ward sometimes. I don't know that I can describe it in words, but I suppose that I could express the mood in terms of an anachronistic mentality resistant to, and protectively ignorant of, any 'unsettling changes' characteristic of, and having lead to the condition of, the world of 1987. (I did in fact hint at this in part 1; perhaps not recognizably so, when I spoke of my feeling on arriving at Willow Walk after an escape; ie, my strong sense of old furniture, and of time having moved backwards.)

One of the dormitories in which I was housed had beds partitioned one from another; ie, as opposed to being open plan, and the man next to me caught my eye by virtue of what I considered at the time was a striking resemblance to Adolf Hitler. I am not now certain in retrospect that I was as convinced that he was indeed Adolf as I was that Anna was Lola, but I must have had some confidence in my theory, for I remember being very keen that my mother should meet him for the sake of world peace; the logic being that, if she could forgive Hitler for World War 2, it would (hopefully) serve the purpose of helping all those of her generation to stop 'living in the past', which I felt they frequently did.

As far as the question of peace in the 'real' world of 1987 was concerned, I don't know that I had any specific policy ideas, even at a very primitive level, but every evening when visitors came and sat around the tables in the dayroom, I felt that it was incumbent upon me to act as a sort of Henry Kissinger. I had an idea that one of these evening visitors was a high ranking Russian diplomat, and another was, I was quite certain, the liberal politician David Steele. (In fact, this individual looked like David Owen, and I'd got the faces muddled, but I still think that the surname Steele sounds more appropriate; don't ask me why.) N.B// (It should perhaps be noted that in fact, I made very little effort to join in these 'round the table discussions'.)

In which I believe that I can cause souls to 'transmigrate' by staring at the T.V., and 'Lola is instrumental in resurrecting Clint'.

I have already mentioned that it was my belief at this time that the reciprocation of my strong feelings for Lola could unite the world, and that the various famous men and women whom I admired could be expected to aid and abet my endeavours in this direction. And I have named Shirley MacLaine as the one celebrity who, to my mind, would be likely to be particularly keen to help me. I did not however, even in spite of my 'high', imagine that Shirley, and others including Clint Eastwood, would simply come waltzing in and 'swear allegiance' to my cause; after all, one of their main attractions as far as I was concerned was their independence of mind and self reliance. And so, in spite of my self belief, and perhaps because of the awe with which I regarded these individuals, I was by no means certain that they would approve of me, or regard my selfish desires as worthy of their time. In fact, just as was the case with Dora, I often felt that Shirley might regard my plight as something I ought to be able to deal with myself and, in classic paranoid fashion, I was frequently fearful that Clint, rather than sympathizing with my position, might take it into his head to shoot me! Nevertheless, whenever I wasn't too restless, I would sit in front of the T.V. in the dayroom and try to 'get them to appear'.

My strongest memory of attempting to 'summon' Shirley MacLaine via the television involves one of

The Total Obliteration Of Hell

the glamorous American soaps; possibly 'Dynasty'. Concentrating my mind, I gazed earnestly at each female face, willing Shirley to appear. As I watched (and I must have had considerable faith that it would work), it seemed to me that each of the females on screen was 'psychically connected to', or 'a version of' Shirley, and that, by a supreme effort of will, I could either replace each actress with a more Shirley-like individual, or else cause the 'Shirleyishness' to be emphasized. And it seemed to be working, for with each new face, I became increasingly convinced that what I was seeing was indeed Ms. MacLaine, heavily disguised. Although I was prepared to 'exercise my power' in this manner, I was not without a certain sense of guilt since, as the seeming indignation on 'Shirley's face' reminded me, in 'forcing souls into and out of bodies and paying no regard to the fate of personality traits not relevant to my summoning', I was surely little less than a murderer. But perhaps the most extreme example of this 'technique' was when I 'got Lola to dig up and resurrect Clint Eastwood' from what looked like the Yorkshire Moors!

I do not as I write this have any clear visual memory of actually 'seeing Lola' on television, either on the occasion that I am about to describe, or at any other time; neither do I recall trying to summon her in the manner in which I endeavoured to 'bring Shirley MacLaine into play'. It is true that on one occasion whilst watching the T.V., I saw a female teacher with long hair who I suspected to be my elusive girlfriend engaged in her work in Madrid, but I think that I realized at least in part that it was just wishful thinking that led me to believe that it was her, even if I didn't admit it to myself at the time. Bearing this in mind, it is hard to convey adequately the sense in which I felt her to be present in what was, I now believe, a feature film version of one of the 'James Herriot' books (about a vet in Yorkshire). Perhaps it was simply that since I wished Lola to be there, so to me she was, and the fact that I didn't recognize her as a visible character was purely academic.

I believe that at the time I was watching the actors who were really present on the moors in this scene, I had already considered the possibility that my macho hero Clint had died of a massive heart attack. (This is probably related to my feeling that in one of his then most recent films; 'Heartbreak Ridge', he had overreached himself in his efforts to keep up physically with the 'increasing madness of the world'; this having taken a heavy toll.) - So, in short, I half thought that Clint was dead and buried: - I sensed that his corpse lay somewhere in the dark basement of a building in what seemed rather like New York. All in all, it is, I must admit, not a little bizarre that I considered that Lola, who I couldn't see, was going to exhume Clint's body (I didn't believe that the 'ultimate hero' could remain lifeless for very long), when 'the body' was on the other side of the Atlantic Ocean! However, it didn't seem problematic to me at the time; digging into peat in Yorkshire seeming as likely a means of triggering the resurrection of Mr. Eastwood as any other. – I was full of admiration for Lola, as I regarded the 'attempted reawakening of Clint from the dead' by her as an act of tremendous courage, since I imagined that he would be none too pleased that his rest had been disturbed. And, in a strange way, I felt that I'd been responsible for his 'death' in the first place. Yes; I was a pathetic coward, who'd messed with things I didn't understand just for the satisfaction of my ego, and, consequently, the world was mad. (I realize that this is in contradiction with things I've said previously about holding answers to the salvation of mankind and retaining the 'lost secret' of love, but then I was full of contradictions. Perhaps the most powerful illustration of my notion of universal responsibility is embodied in my balmy idea that I'd caused the sun to shrink; either that, or caused the earth to recede from it.)

Frank Hayward

In which I think that I may have caused the sun to shrink, and am concerned that my head may explode

Quite how I came to regard the disk of the sun as smaller than was customary I have no inkling; after all, I'd looked at it a million times before, and so ought to have been extremely familiar with its apparent size. And as to when I first perceived that it was 'smaller than usual', I have no recollection. I vividly remember how aware I was that it was 'unusually tiny' whilst on a rare (at that time) visit to the hospital shop (possibly in early May of 1987), but I am certain that, by that time, my concern regarding this matter was already well established, since I also recall being somewhat relieved when the reddening disk had looked as large as I felt it ought to one evening about Easter time: - I believe that it was on the evening of the Easter (1987) hospital disco. – It was also my concern that, whether as a result of a modification of the earth's orbit, or for some other reason, the direction of the sunrise was 'wrong', and one morning (possibly on a day in March or April), I spent quite some time attempting to 'coax' the sun to rise where it 'ought to'. Furthermore, if I remember correctly, I believe that I was even worried that instead of one sun rising, two might quite possibly appear: - things were that messed up!

Quite why I felt that I had to bear (or even consider the possibility of bearing) responsibility for such potential disasters on the cosmic scale, once again

The Total Obliteration Of Hell

I don't know that I can adequately explain; I certainly have no firm convictions regarding this subject, but perhaps it could be related to my feeling that I was the centre of my universe. That I considered myself in these terms is (arguably) well illustrated by another of the rather fantastic and disturbing ideas which had a hold on me at this time; namely that my head was, in a sense, a planet. (I have already referred to my morbid fantasy about my head 'shattering like an exploding planet'.) As to how I regarded this 'planet head' of mine as relating to the larger earth I don't know that I even considered, so it is perhaps difficult to be sure whether the fear of 'assassination' by being shot in the head that came upon me every so often, and the even more 'inspiring' urge to break into a mad dash in order to leap into space like 'Superman' and leave the larger sphere behind me, related to a conviction that the wider world was under threat of destruction (perhaps as a consequence of actions and/or thoughts of mine?), or simply to a 'humbler' paranoia regarding my personal safety, but perhaps both strands were present?; at all events, both fears were of things that would amount to the same result; i.e. planet earth being 'in jeopardy' 'threatened my life', and so did 'being subject to the murderous intentions of an anonymous sniper': - either way, I was doomed to be blasted to oblivion! But these feelings were transient, and occupied relatively small portions of my days.

Frank Hayward

On Shirley MacLaine

I have made a number of references to the American actress/dancer (she is many things) Shirley MacLaine, and indicated that I felt that there was a strong bond between her and myself. This is no 'wacky', flash-in-the-pan feeling, but a longstanding conviction from pre mental illness days, that is undiminished even as I write. To me, 'Shirley's universe' embraces everything that I value in life, and her autobiographical writings have acted as the perfect catalyst to stimulate the opening of my mind and heart. And in 1987, so impressed was I by the idea of Shirley's insatiable curiosity about, and apparently inexhaustible ability to appreciate, and draw inspiration from, everything animal, vegetable and mineral, and everything beyond the realms of the visible, that I coined the term 'Maclaining' for all enthusiastically pursued activity, and chose to regard myself, on those occasions that I was not too carried away by my own supposed importance, as a sort of 'poor version' of Shirley, who would hopefully not 'stain the MacLaine name'.

However, as I indicated when I referred to my fear of Shirley and myself physically colliding, I was not without a certain degree of anxiety for the fate of her unparalleled (to my way of thinking) questioning intelligence, and I often felt that she was very likely going quite mad herself, or, as I put it at the time, had been 'sent back to nursery school'. (This was based on the notion that her mind was not unlike mine, and that she too had bitten off more than she could chew from the 'tree of knowledge'.) But I was not without hope that, had she indeed reverted to infancy or childhood, her sheer doggedness would win through, and she would rapidly break through the walls of the mind prison into which she had fallen and reassume her place as the world's 'number one solid gold actress': - I frequently pictured her in a gold sequined stage outfit.

However, and whether through an intellectually competitive streak in my own ego I'm not sure, I was still dubious about the basis of Shirley's wisdom; ie, was tender love supreme, or was she motivated more by a drive to succeed and understand and be empowered by all that was around her even at the expense (through ignorance) of the one quality that she'd always (perhaps unwittingly?) inspired me to regard as paramount? (It is true that I'm writing this now having read her most recent autobiographies, in which she herself speaks of her wish to become more closely aligned with her 'feminine side', so it might be that I'm trying to take credit for her own realizations about the shortcomings of power and aggressiveness, untempered by the non-judgementalness and patient appreciation of yielding love. However, even if I am in fact grafting what is expressed in Shirley's most recent writings onto my genuine memories of 1987, my attempt at accurately representing what I remember of my thoughts is a sincere one.)

Frank Hayward

On saving the world with Shirley, Clint and Peter

Whilst having referred to my notion that various celebrities would/might quite possibly come to my aid, and that this would somehow lead to Lola and myself being united, and the world, or indeed the universe, being 'saved', or successfully 'completed' by the magic of our 'great love', I have not as yet spoken of the means by which I considered this might be achieved, as and when Shirley etc should arrive on the scene. However, in saying this, I guess that I'm no better than a sensation seeking journalist, since (and I'm sure that it comes as no great surprise) I had no clearly formulated notion of the steps I felt would be required to achieve this desired end, besides which, I had no fixed vision of the 'happy ever after' in which Lola and myself would reside. – But I was not entirely without fantasies as to the means and the specifics of the nature of the final goal.

As far as the 'getting there' aspect was concerned, I had a mental picture of Shirley and myself in an old, hired car, driving about looking for clues that might help solve the riddles of 'life, the universe and everything', and at the same time, sort out the 'hiccough' in my love life; ie, deal with the unrequited aspect of my love for Lola. But, as was/is characteristic of the fancy idea I have of my personality, I saw a possible 'spanner in the works'; namely that Shirley might discover that Lola was not intended to be 'the girl for me', and that I would have to choose between my wish to seek out truth,

The Total Obliteration Of Hell

and to live accordingly, and remaining stubbornly devoted to the 'doomed concept' of Lola and myself; an alternative which would probably reflect my stubbornness more than any genuine feeling I had for the 'poor girl'!

Curiously enough, another famous face whose aid I imagined being accessible to me was someone with whose stance regarding questions of spirituality and religious philosophy I was by no means well informed.

I can currently identify four reasons as to why the highly individual rock star and former 'Genesis' front man Peter Gabriel appealed to me as ideal for the job; (1) I had previously known a girl who had claimed to have been on first name terms with said Peter; (2) 'The Lamb Lies Down On Broadway' (in many ways the seminal Genesis album) seemed (and perhaps even seems) to be based on life transforming events either analogous to, or directly to do with, the experience of mental illness; (3) the name Gabriel symbolized religiosity; and (4) (and not leastly) I was sure that one of the night nurses was none other than Mr. Gabriel himself. (As far as this last point is concerned, there was in fact very little similarity in appearance between the two, but once the face of the nurse in question was stamped on my brain, it appeared to belong to the 'genuine article'.)

Perhaps because 'Peter' was frequently on duty and therefore in sight, 'his' role was even more on my mind than that of Shirley with regard to 'healing the world', added to which, I may also have felt that he was, if not as intelligent as Shirl', probably purer and better informed when it came to the essential nature of reality, being 'not many steps below Jesus' on the 'cosmic scale'. (I think that I felt I was becoming quite a cosmic socialite!) – However, in spite of my tremendous admiration for the magnificence of 'Mr. Gabriel', I felt no shame or inferiority at being in such 'Godly company' since, whilst not imagining myself to be Jesus, I was adamant that I had 'realized my place in the nature of all things'; I 'was' 'King Frank of Narnia', and not to be messed with! (I regarded my relationship with Peter Gabriel as not dissimilar to that between 'Richard the Lionheart' (me) and 'Robin Hood' (him).)

'Peter's' west country accent was further 'evidence' that the nurse in question was indeed he, since my long lost friend Kathy Grammer had spoken of discovering a recording studio near Bath that belonged to Gabriel. In this vein, I concocted the paranoid fantasy that 'Peter'; or Philip (as he liked to be called) was not quite as holy as he appeared, and was in fact the driving force behind the 'subversive goings on' at night at the hospital; namely that patients were being drugged up and fed so as to be fattened up. I hardly dared to imagine what possible sinister purpose this action was intended to promote, but it certainly didn't seem to be in our best interests. And another awful possibility was in the forefront of my mind for some time; namely that, when I'd first met my 'precious' Lola in England, she'd latched onto me not out of friendship, but because she was in fact employed by the hospital to 'hook' young men and women; ie, her job being to draw them into the 'drug culture' of the Psychy' Unit, from which escape, if possible, was unlikely.

Perhaps strangely, I didn't torture myself over the idea that I had been betrayed, but it did raise the exciting possibility that 'my' Lola was, unbeknownst to me, almost permanently resident in England, 'plying her iniquitous trade'; perhaps as close as Trent Park.* (It was presumably for this reason that I set forth one evening for Trent Park disco: - see later.)

In spite of my reservations about Philip the night nurse; and I have not mentioned the fact that he had 'had to' force feed me my medication one night (I had at the time thought that he was trying to strangle me), I was sufficiently full of my own supposed importance that I little doubted my ability to take advantage of his 'superstar status'. And I suppose I also felt that, once he realized that I had been friendly with Ms. Grammer, he would be full of remorse for his rough treatment, and only too willing to offer me the skill of 'Rael', the hero of 'The Lamb'.

Philip would often come and go at a run, and when the radio played 'his' songs, I would imagine him off somewhere halfway round the globe doing his bit for world peace, or 'bounding about' in my bedroom at Willow Walk, examining my philosophical writings, and leaving me presents befitting my 'kingly status', and by way of penance for 'half strangling me to death' as I put it: - clearly this had occurred before he'd realized how 'special' I was!

Since first hearing one of the early Genesis albums, I had had the impression that Peter (Gabriel) was disenchanted with 'the almighty', since one of the lyrics referred to God having abandoned the earth long ago: - what if the 'Messenger of the Lord' were to have a resurgence of faith – surely this would mean a great deal for the human race? And surely my 'unique' belief in love would trigger just such a revival? (I must however admit that, in accordance with my doubts about my purity of motive, I was not entirely sure that my potential influence on such a 'noble' figure as Peter might not lead to his corruption by way of inspiring him to false prophecy and, by so doing, seal my fate as the lowest of the low even more decisively than had my past actions).

A third 'giant figure' from whom I suspected aid might be forthcoming was of course Clint, although I saw his potential function as rather different from that of the other two; he was to be 'St. Mathew – the Antichrist'! Quite why I should have decided that the Apostle Mathew was the 'Antichrist' I cannot imagine, but that Clint should be a dark and destructive element seemed appropriate enough, for if someone had to play the part, who better than 'Dirty Harry', or 'the man with no name'; who else could cope with such a thankless occupation as being as it were diametrically opposed to J.C. without dissolving in a blubbering mass of shame and guilt?! (My limited understanding of eastern mysticism inclined me to believe that there had to be a counter to the positive purity of Jesus in order for there to be balance in the cosmos. I suppose that 'the Devil' would have done, but I regarded an actual Satan as a myth. - I should add that I didn't consider Clint to be 'evil'; just necessary.)

* I believe that by this time, my conviction that Anna was Lola had faded.

Frank Hayward

A vague notion of a world that has been saved

Proceeding to my fantasy vision of the paradise that I 'would' eventually occupy with my true love, I am at once aware, now that I come to write about it, just how little I had actually envisioned life in my 'brave new world' beyond its inception. I have already referred to my wishing to wake up in my own bed to find that paradise had appeared overnight, and with Lola by my bedside to reassure me that I really had 'died for love'. However, beyond fantasies of going downstairs for a celebratory breakfast whilst revelling in the peaceful, sunny morning (cars would have been banished), and watching joyous celebrations of the end of the old world on T.V., and further dreamy notions concerning the slightly less immediate future that everyone would go on dream holidays with their loved ones for as long as they liked, and enjoy picnics (on which I would consume platefuls of chicken sandwiches), it did not seem necessary to consider things further; beauty and joy proceeding to blossom beyond imagination. (I believe that I had, by 1987, read C.S. Lewis's 'The Last Battle', which describes the coming of paradise in this manner.)

Perhaps these idle dreams were more telling than I knew, in that they reflected my predilection with aspects of the known physical universe and the experience of sensation; ie, as if, were the world to appear to be paradise, and everyone around me to appear happy, then that would be paradise or, to put it another way, I focussed on ideas of a world externally perfect as bringing bliss rather than considering the quality of mind required to appreciate a heaven or nirvana. Of course, that is not in any way to suggest that I did not regard peace of mind as an intrinsic part of the deal. It may also be worth noting my emphasis on the perpetuation of many aspects of life on earth as I had known it up to that point. Perhaps this is a positive reflection of my feeling that the world had been a wonderful place in many ways, and that I had no wish for more than the joys that I'd found in nature and material comforts, but it could be said, and perhaps I'm not 'spiritually qualified' to speak on the subject, that these feelings are more noteworthy for being indicators of my attachment to all that I had associated with happiness (however genuine the happiness), and which I had in a way deified, thereby confusing 'the wood' with 'the trees'.

Frank Hayward

Love/hate

Whilst I have said that I didn't literally believe in the existence of 'the Devil', there is no question that both my periods of psychosis involved viewing particular people as either all good or bad, or at least predominantly one or the other. However, it is certainly not the case that, having once been convinced that a particular individual was a 'thoroughly bad lot', I would maintain my view unshakeably, or that I was entirely incapable of seeing anything in other than black and white terms. Perhaps the best example of my love/hate, and positions in between, concerns my feelings towards my mother during the first six months of 1987.

I will not reiterate the drama of the night I 'died'; if it is not fresh in the reader's mind then I would refer him or her back to the relevant pages. Looking at my written impressions of that evening, it is clear that my feelings towards my mother were unequivocally hostile. As I return in my mind to that period, it seems to me that I felt my hatred to be perfectly natural, on the basis that I was sure that she intended to do me harm. That I felt that way I have no doubt, for I remember being in our kitchen one afternoon/evening, and watching mother like a hawk, or, more accurately, like a sparrow that is watching a hawk; imagining that I was in danger of being stabbed by her with a kitchen knife. And I also clearly recall telling her; although I may in fact have kept the thought to myself, that she was in

The Total Obliteration Of Hell

truth a particular French girl who had poisoned her parents; this being based on a mental association between my mother's 'violet-blue' eyes and the name of this girl; Violette. But there was an additional reason why I found it impossible to think well of mum at this time, relating to my relationship to her as dependent son; this manifested itself in what might be described as a mild psychosomatic pain causing me discomfort at the base of my spine that I associated with a pull that I felt her body had on me: - as she moved in front of me, her behind seemed to be drawing me towards her as if there was a force bonding me to her.* In view of my paranoia, it is perhaps not surprising that I was convinced that she was aware of what she was doing; ie, I believed that she was deliberately causing me physical discomfort by her movements. Perhaps I felt that this reflected a possessiveness of me; whatever, I was certain that she used this 'trick' as a means by which to punish, and exert power over, me. (I do not remember for certain whether this unpleasant sensation ceased on the night that I 'broke free' and 'died', but I am certain that it didn't last for more than a week or two.) Bearing in mind the intensity of the resentment and suspicion that I bore towards mum at this time, my reactions to her presence may, if not supported, at least be understood; i.e., I acted as though I had disowned her and; and I cannot remember on how many occasions, punched her arms: - and legs?

Allied to the notion I had that, like it or not, I could not get 'out of her clutches', I was convinced that mother would do anything in her power to terminate my friendship with Lola and, although much of the time she (mum) spoke little to me; presumably because she was worried that it might antagonize me further, we did actually have a two-way row on this subject, that blew up because I'd lost the last letter that Lola had sent me, and (of course) thought that mum had taken it. In the course of this contretemps, I believe that I tried to assert my 'revolutionary position', and, presumably, although I don't remember my particular line, strove desperately to make clear that my affiliation lay with my 'girlfriend', and that I wouldn't stand for any attempt to harm or abort my relationship with her.

The fact of my being taken back into Chase Farm on January 16th must have been a godsend as far as mum was concerned, and from my point of view offered the perfect opportunity to seek a 'genuinely caring replacement' for the woman who I felt had either simply ceased to care, or had (perhaps) never been concerned with my welfare. One of the 'replacements' was Dora (and anyone more epitomizing the 'mother goddess' would have been hard to find), but she was somehow too much of a 'universal mother' to be for me alone, and 'much too cosmically important'. Whether I consciously sought out someone else I'm not sure, but my 'new mother' soon materialized in a pink dressing gown and, for a short space, Esme Hayward receded to the sidelines, although I believe that I thought of her now and then, and imagined her 'swanning around with her well-heeled friends' whilst my father patiently suffered on Napier Ward.

The Total Obliteration Of Hell

As to whether Imelda's mother chose to regard me as some kind of surrogate son I am not sure, but I may have thought that she did, if only fleetingly, and the thought may have been influential in prompting my 'adoption' of her as my 'new mum'. I can cite three other possibly influential factors in this regard; namely, (1) since Imelda seemed like a version of Lola, her mother thus seemed akin to my true love; (2) she (Imelda's mother) seemed inconsolably upset, which was in stark contrast with the 'scheming frivolity' of my biological mother; and (3) she gave me a small token (a key I think) which I took to be a sign that she felt that we had a common bond. As I reflect, a fourth possible factor or reason comes to mind; namely that she said something about me that I interpreted as complimentary: - perhaps this is a more pertinent explanation. (I ought to stress that I was not all that clear about anything that she said, which is hardly surprising, since neither of us was in a particularly fit state to converse, and English was not her first language.) A further reason that I wished to 'swop' my mother may have been that 'Frank Hayward' was 'dead', and 'I' needed a new life.

It may be that I have overstated the extent to which I acted independently of my maternal blood tie, for I remember phoning mother several times from the payphone on Suffolk Ward; unprovoked as it were by any message from her. As far as I can recall, the 'issue' concerning me, and prompting the phone calls, was my paranoid fear that my life was in danger from the ward staff; my thinking being that my mother was someone who had influence, and that it was possible that she could step in to save me if she so wished. And I certainly intended to survive, and was quite prepared to swallow my pride and employ all options or, more accurately, my only option: - the 'crafty, crazy Mrs. Hayward'! It need hardly be added that said individual did not seem overenthusiastic about 'halting my demise'; - I put it down to her having her head buried in the sand, or possibly wishing to be rid of me behind a painted facade of patronizing ignorance as to my likely fate, concealing infuriated indignation that I should trouble her with such a 'minor matter' as whether I should live or die! (It is clear that I was getting over 'being dead' very quickly; either that or else that I considered myself to be both dead and yet still capable of being killed?)

Mum didn't visit me at all for the first few weeks of my stay on Suffolk Ward. On reflection, I can hardly blame her if it was simply a matter of choice not to come on her part, but she maintains that, with my father's worsening condition and her various responsibilities, it was not a question of having decided that she didn't wish to see me. I believe that when she did finally show up, I was so bowled over by how glamorous she looked (my 'solid gold, Shirley MacLaine mum'), and so pleased with the chocolate bars and wine gums she showered on me, that all I could think of was making the most of her presence (and presents). However, once she'd gone, I don't doubt that I pretty quickly decided that I'd been no more than one of her 'charity calls', and that she'd not stayed a minute longer than she could help. And so, in spite of the fact that I enjoyed what seemed almost a royal visit, and readily reverted to my former dependence on mother for comfort and security, and despite a surge of pride at her social skills and good looks (and I was actually aware that I was proud of her), I did not so readily relinquish the idea that, basically, what I was seeing was no more than a show of good manners for the sake of the self satisfaction she would gain by fulfilling her 'maternal duty' and charming everyone who saw her. I suppose that my antipathy was sustained to a certain extent by comparing her with my father, who I was tending to regard by this time as some sort of saint as I envisioned him wasting away, seamlessly stoical and without complaint: - selfless in fact.

I don't believe that I considered dad to be actually 'at the mercy' of my mother during his final few weeks at home; ie, after having left Napier Ward; but his 'emptiness' seemed far removed from the 'ebullience' and 'calculating cleverness' of the other. So fixed was I in my mind that mum was as I considered her to be; ie, full of herself and her popularity in her social world, that it came as quite a revelation when, during one of my 'breakouts', I witnessed a far less showy individual, who was quietly considerate and unselfconsciously concerned with the care of her dying husband. It was as if all the 'artifice' and 'social splendour' were designed out of a very private modesty that sought to convince the world that she was as shallow as I'd thought, and suddenly I felt that she was an unsung heroine upon whom my father was pathetically reliant.

I would be lying were I to say that this 'fresh insight' into mother revolutionized my attitude towards her, or that it marked a turning point at which I decided that I had been unfairly judgmental of her. And besides, as far as accepting once more that she was my mum and I her son was concerned, I'd probably already done so by that time although, once again, I'm lost with regard to the chronological sequence of events during this period. But there is no doubt that the harshness of my attitude softened by degrees, since by about May of 1987 I was impersonating mum's voice to myself (and to anyone who happened to be listening) and, whilst such behaviour may not be indicative of an 'appropriate reverence', it does at least suggest that I was once again able to think of her idiosyncrasies without simply 'seeing red'.

Having suggested that my changing attitude to my mother was the clearest example of the 'blackness and whiteness' of my feelings and their inconsistency, it strikes me that my feelings towards my father were at least equally powerful either way at different times; ie, in '85 he'd 'been the Devil', whereas, as he lay dying so I'd 'made him' a saint. But I will not go into this, since it would involve much repetition of earlier parts of my tale: - a sufficiently dedicated reader could always pursue the subject by referring to the relevant pages.

* I have already mentioned a slight pain at the base of my spine; this was an identical pain; ie, although I have associated the ache with the presence of my

mother, I was also aware of it sometimes when not in her company.

Frank Hayward

On my (limited) relationships whilst in hospital
during my second period of psychosis

Whether it comes across in what I've written I don't
know (and I have not consciously striven to see that
it should), but it strikes me as I reflect upon it now,
that 'my world' in hospital in 1987, whilst having
been 'large' on powerful sensations, impressions
and concerns, was very short on relationships with
others, even at a very superficial and/or deluded
level. This may, and perhaps should, come as no
surprise considering my mental state, but it might
nevertheless be regarded as worthy of note,
especially by comparison with the situation during
the spring of '85, when I at least had, and was
capable of appreciating, the comradeship of Kevin,
Diane, and to a lesser extent Gelli and Joey.
However, although such an observation is quite in
line with my long held view that I was 'even
madder' in '87 than was the case on the earlier
occasion, it might be misleading to suppose that my
relative lack of 'playmates' this time around reflects
a relatively greater 'disintegration of my
personality'; ie, rather than simply being
symptomatic of there being fewer suitable people
on the ward in '87 with whom I could share a
common bond. But of course, the fact that I have
not really spoken of friendships in part 2 does not in
itself necessarily mean that I was devoid of
companionship. But there is I must admit, little
doubt in my mind that the spring of '87 was not for
me a time memorable for friendships; I was far too
wrapped up in, and excited by, my ceaseless

interpretation of people and events: - in short, my life was like a film which I was merely watching, rather than being on screen.

Amongst those people with whom I could be said to communicate (as opposed to those who made a particularly powerful impression on me, but with whom I shared little in the way of conversation), pride of place ought perhaps be given to the nurses who were assigned to my personal care, or more cynically, given the task of ensuring that I didn't get out of order. (Because I was pretty crazy at this time, it is not possible for me to state with certainty the precise role prescriptions of any of these nurses and student nurses, or even to be sure that my belief that they were all assigned specifically to me at any time was in fact the case.)

Karin

Karin was a student nurse; possibly older than some of them, but certainly less than thirty, and possibly only apparently older by virtue of her seriousness, and a tiredness in her voice and face that suggested world weariness. Looking back on what must have been considerable tolerance on her part, I almost regret that I didn't take more advantage of her thoughtful and attentive concern, but it is probably as well that I didn't become enamoured of her, and that I tended to regard her rather as some sort of female reporter who had been sent to spend some time with a flamboyant celebrity. It may be far fetched to regard her as having been someone with whom I had much of a staff/patient relationship but, having seen her since during a visit to the Casualty Department, when she reminded me of the occasion upon which I flooded my bedroom floor by overfilling the wash basin (Karin had apparently requested that I take a shower), it would perhaps be mean not to give her a mention. Besides, I must confess to loving the idea that she remembers me as someone who had a certain 'je ne sais quoi'!

The Total Obliteration Of Hell

Michael

Michael was another nurse (although not a student) who I remember as being rather long suffering. This was conveyed in part by his throaty voice, and also by a rather melancholy facial expression. However, this latter characteristic may simply have been a reaction to my behaviour each time we were in close proximity, since I would tell him that he had leprosy, but that I was a great faith healer and could cure him! As might perhaps be expected, Michael was not over the moon at my diagnosis, and protested that the marks on his neck were the result of a rash: - I dismissed his explanation as ignorance. As with Karin, it is debatable that I mention him at all, since our communication did not extend beyond the confines of this frequently enacted scene for some time. However, and maybe because I knew him during the latter part of my 'sentence', and the 'high tide' of my insanity was just about on the turn, he slowly won my trust to a degree, and was even able to give me a shave without my fearing for my life. (I had thought him to be a black 'Charles Bronson', out to kill me in the blink of an eye, but by now I'd realized that he was just a 'big softee'!)

Steve

Steve was another student who either volunteered to take me under his wing or was instructed to do so. Being male, and about my age, and having an easy going manner, whilst not lacking in the self possession appropriate to his position of responsibility, he was well placed to take advantage of my slowly returning lucidity. My happiest memory of my acquaintance with Steve is of when he took me for a walk to the nurses' homes and permitted me to see his room, offering me a glass of blackcurrant or something similar. It was a welcome change from the ward and, although I had always got a big kick out of escaping, it was good to feel that for once I was outside without being a fugitive. Whether this outing marked a significant point in my rehabilitation I am not sure, but I considered Steve's action to have been a great kindness, even though I was slightly unsettled when I saw his personal possessions, for they looked rather familiar; ie, compare with the sense I'd had in Shona's room that she had somehow gotten hold of Lola's things. However, on this occasion, the insecurity was directed towards my stuff at Willow Walk. I suppose that my rationale was that Steve had got hold of some of this, so I reasoned that my paintings and writings and all my accumulated treasures were highly vulnerable to the 'predations' of anyone who called at our house.

The Total Obliteration Of Hell

Some other staff and patients with whom I interrelated.

There are a number of other members of staff with whom I developed the tiniest inkling of a rapport, if I can use such a strong word without misleading the reader into supposing that more than the flimsiest of understandings came to exist between them and myself.

Our 'relationships' hardly merit going into, but I would like to show that I appreciated the company of these people by mentioning them by name: - Jean; Anna; Carol; Carolyn; Goodie; Tina the cleaner; 'Nessie', and Tony. As regards those patients with whom I had a friendly acquaintance, I would mention Pauline; a very pleasant, slim, and impeccably dressed lady in her mid forties who I tried to coax into walking along the corridor because she seemed to be rooted to the spot, and with whom I subsequently developed a very unstrained acquaintance; Alan, in spite of his breaking my spectacles; Stephen, in spite of his trying to force me to go back to bed because, or so he told me, Sam didn't want to see me up and about; Maria, who had a very warm, if somewhat earthy, personality, and who seemed quite the sanest of people; and Eileen, who I didn't know very well, but who kindly gave me an Easter egg. – Two other patients; Gelli, who I have already mentioned in connection with my first time in Chase Farm; and Philip Hooker, must also be accounted for, since I had quite a lot to do with them in '87, but can hardly be considered as having been friends due to the severity of their illnesses.

The Total Obliteration Of Hell

Mr. Hayward 'on the loose'!

I have no idea as to the number of times that I made a bid for freedom during my enforced stay in hospital in 1987, but there is no question that a very large proportion of these attempts were pathetically unsuccessful, by which I mean to say that I didn't even make it out of the building. In fact, it would probably be true to say that 8 or 9 times out of 10 I was intercepted by the staff. (This proportion very likely increased with each attempt, as it became more and more obvious that I couldn't be trusted to resist any opportunity to try and 'spread my wings'.) I would also not like to hazard a guess as to the number of times I got as far as the open air, but was caught whilst still inside the hospital grounds. However, on those occasions on which I actually reached the outside world (this can only have been a handful of times), I seldom failed to reach my destination. This, as might be expected, was usually Willow Walk. But that is not to say that I invariably either managed to enter, or spend any appreciable time inside, the house. For a start, if I didn't have a door key with me and rang the bell, I ran the risk of being recognized through the translucent glass of the front door, or of having the door opened and closed again (when I was identified) too quickly for me to force my way in. Furthermore, if I was able to gain access with a key but was spotted before having had time to reach my bedroom, it was often my fate to be requested to leave. (My mentally-handicapped brother Tim was particularly disturbed by these intrusions.) I don't remember ever being physically thrown out of the house: - sometimes, my other brother Peter said he'd drive me back to the ward and, whether out of fear or respect or something else, I tended to give in. Another ploy, used by my mother, was to threaten to call the police; this sometimes had sufficient deterrent effect, but on at least one occasion I had to be coaxed out of my bedroom by uniformed officers. On the way back to Chase Farm in their van (or whatever), I showed them my favourite coloured slide of Lola! I don't remember what I said about her to them, or their reaction.

The Total Obliteration Of Hell

Escape to Trent Park in search of Lola

I have already touched upon the fact that one of my 'illicit pedestrian adventures' had as its intended destination Trent Park disco, and suggested that the purpose of the trip was to satisfy my burning curiosity about whether Lola would be there: - I pictured her in my mind's eye as she had appeared when she had been in England in 1982. And I also said that I suspected that she might have been somehow responsible for my having landed up in Chase Farm in the first place. Perhaps this delusion was a distorted reflection of what may have been closer to the truth; ie, that my craziness was tied up with my obsession with her. (I cannot emphasize too strongly that I do not now hold her in any way responsible for my insanity; yes, she may have unwittingly served as a catalyst for my 'downfall', but only because I was 'ripe' for it; ie, to blame her would be like blaming a hot sun for causing one to sweat. In other words, I only suffered from Lola's honesty because I hadn't learned to deal with my infatuation, and expected her to simply fit in with my deluded notions of love.) But I must return to the matter at hand; namely, the daring perambulation I took one evening; quite possibly a Wednesday or a Friday, these being the nights on which the disco had been held at the time I regularly frequented it.

It is unfortunate that I cannot remember for certain whether I was dressed in my pyjamas on this occasion, as it might help to evoke the scene more precisely. However, to the best of my belief, I had an overcoat, possibly covering a stripy dressing gown and pyjamas and, somewhat incredibly, as will become clear when I describe the terrain, nothing but loosely fitting regulation foam slippers, with socks, on my feet. (I'm quite sure about the foam slippers, because I recall leaving one behind in the mud.) Quite why I chose to journey 'cross country' I'm not absolutely clear, but it may have been because (a), it seemed bolder and more romantic; (b), because it was a more direct route; or (c) (and perhaps more significantly), because I felt that it would reduce my chances of being intercepted or having to pass any strangers: - I was quite paranoid. Without looking it up, I am not sure of the name of the farm that I had to pass on leaving the road about half a mile from the hospital, but it is probably not important, especially as I doubt that I was aware of it at the time.

It is hard to convey the immensity of the insecurity I felt as I marched 'bravely' along Hadley Road, trying desperately to appear as 'normal' as possible, but the magnitude of my fear of discovery may be gauged by the fact that rather than risk barking dogs and an irate farmer as a consequence of taking the access road, I chose instead to stumble through a hedge. Once in the fields I continued to stumble, breathing heavily and making clumsy progress in my nervously excited haste and ill chosen footwear. The vast sky (it had never seemed so big to me) was a glaring orange (the reflection of suburban London's sodium lights on the uniform cloud), but it seemed to me that its appearance was to be accounted for by the

The Total Obliteration Of Hell

'madness' of the universe: - I believe that I thought that the absence of stars was a consequence of the 'mess we were in', rather than having to do with the weather.

I don't believe that I had had the foresight to bring much, or any, tobacco with me but, although I stopped now and then to survey the way ahead, and either smoked what I had or else bemoaned my lack of this substance, I was not deflected from my purpose, and pressed on across a muddy field (I think that it had been ploughed) until I came upon a swollen stream. This was not entirely unexpected. I'm not sure if I leaped across or found a bridge, but I was not detained for long, and pretty soon stood at the boundary of the woods between myself and the college. I thought of Shona, who was on leave from the ward at that time; she would surely squeal with delight if she knew what I was about: - I'd have a tale to tell alright! However, my unbalanced mind was fearful of the quaking ground hereabouts, and the possibility that, were I to step accidentally in a large puddle, I might be sucked down into the bowels of the earth. In view of my fears, I trod very gingerly, and continued to do so on entering the shadowy world beneath the trees, further terrified that I might step on or otherwise awaken horrific mutant creatures that had (possibly) evolved in what I considered to have become the chaos of creation! Luckily for me, the moon appeared. I cannot remember at precisely what point this occurred, even supposing that I registered it, but it had certainly done so by the time I had come in sight of the Trent Park lakes, since the lower one;

in which I had planned to end my life the previous year, was shining silverily. I was filled with romance, and wondered whether to dive into its depths, though not now to drown myself, but to 'prove my love' for Lola!

As I approached the college, I could hear the voices of students, and I probably wondered whether I'd be challenged before I was able to reach the disco. – There was no one manning the entrance to the students' union bar, where the discos were (and still are I believe) held, but once inside, I was soon approached by a young woman, who either wanted to know if I was a student, or if, student or not, I had a ticket. I'm not sure what I said in reply; I don't believe I was carrying any money, and I certainly had no ticket. However, after a few moments, she let me be.

I'm not sure that I did in fact make a particularly thorough investigation of the premises in order to ascertain whether Lola was present, but I did ask a group of strangers if they'd seen Keith Broadbent (my psychologist friend). Strange to say, since I had no reason to suppose that they knew who he was (it did not strike me at the time as odd to ask these unfamiliar people), I was sure that one of them said that he'd just left, and this piece of information irritated me, I think because it suggested to me that, had he (Keith) been 'psychically in tune', he would have realized that we were intended to meet there. - I don't know how long I stayed at the disco, but I remember that I danced a little, and surveyed the jukebox. I have

The Total Obliteration Of Hell

said that I believed that I had no cash with me, but perhaps I did have a little change, because I tried to get 'Don't Give Up', by Peter Gabriel and Kate Bush, to play, but maybe I thought that I could achieve this without payment? Whatever, I'm sure that this song was played at some stage, because I recall thinking that Peter and Kate sounded dismayed, which inclined me to suppose that they were angry with me for having somehow abused my 'newly discovered spirituality'; ie, I was a fake and a false prophet, and notwithstanding their deeply compassionate natures, they were repelled by my wish to associate with them.

At length I left the bar; perhaps I was bored, and wandered about outside, intrigued by some sort of wire structure in the car park which was shrouded in mist. I believe that I was contemplating heading for Willow Walk when I was caught in the light of a torch beam.

I don't remember my reply to the question posed by the security man, or for that matter what his line was, but he was unhesitant in ushering me into his office: - perhaps this was in part related to my curious appearance? My reaction to the closed circuit television in the office was to become convinced that my supposed notoriety was finally to be rewarded; ie, I was sure that I would soon be appearing on the news. The office wall was adorned by full face, passport-style photographs of what I naturally assumed to be students: - it still seems to me to have been a reasonable assumption. I'm not sure why, although I didn't consider it odd at the time, but all the faces appeared to be female, and it struck me, as I scanned the prints, that my behaviour might be interpreted as indicative of paedophile tendencies (this was perhaps irrational considering the likely age of the girls), but at the time, I really didn't give a damn! – In due course, I was driven back to Chase; I don't recall who by: - I do distinctly remember thinking during the journey about the Black Cuillin mountains of the Isle of Skye, and may have proffered a remark on the subject to my 'chauffeur'. Upon my return, Philip was waiting for me; I think that he had softened towards me by this time; he referred to me as his 'old mate' in his strong regional accent. – It is not I don't suppose of any consequence, but my memory of the location of the room in which I slept that night is that it was not in the Psychy' Unit, but I was probably simply disorientated.

(Slightly later in the year; about May time?, I took another 'excursion' to Trent Park; this time in daylight. My intention on this occasion was to show up for work at the prefab where I'd been employed until January 15th. I managed to accomplish the journey, once again cross country, but although none of my colleagues said anything to my face, it was soon obvious even to me that I was not considered to be in a fit state to do more than permit myself to be humoured by them.)

The Total Obliteration Of Hell

Escape by bus

In addition to escaping to Willow Walk and Trent Park, there was, to the best of my memory, one further location that I reached beyond the confines of the hospital; this time by public transport, although this destination (Edmonton Green) was not actually intended.

I had decided that the reality of 1987 was very different from that of the past. I still considered that everything supposedly unusual about the planet and beyond had been instigated on the fateful night of my return on the ferry from Holland two years previously. I'm not sure how I accounted for the apparent normality of the period following my first breakdown; ie, prior to the resumption of my 'strange thoughts'; - I suppose that I simply dismissed this interlude as an insignificant lapse into a hankering for a past that no longer actually existed. At all events, the 'reality' of the present had a much stronger pull, and my experiences of early 1985 seemed much more akin to what I was now going through. – In the present context; ie, as far as this relates to the unauthorized bus ride that I took one day during the late spring of 1987 I was, to a degree, convinced that, were I to board a bus (any bus), I would be taken to Willow Walk. And I was also fairly certain that the journey would not involve payment. (I suppose that it could be said that both of these beliefs related to my presumption of power and 'specialness', but it would be wrong I think to ignore my then current notion that such things as bus routes, and payment/non payment for using buses, had both been markedly affected by the 'change in reality' that everything and everyone had undergone.) (N.B// It was also a belief of mine that I could convince the driver of any vehicle leaving the hospital car park to take me home by telling them how urgent it was that I got there. Perhaps it is fortunate that I did not put this theory to the test.) – But I must revert to the simple telling of the tale although, in this instance, there is not much to tell.

Having made my way to the front entrance of the hospital, I boarded a bus without paying; hurriedly climbing the staircase and taking up a position at the front of the top deck. I have three abiding memories of the journey. Firstly, I was hyperconscious of seemingly being literally on top of the traffic in front and of the limited width of the road, and was quite certain that there would be a collision with another vehicle. Secondly, it seemed to me inevitable that any pedestrians crossing in front of the bus would be run over. The third lasting impression; also indicative of a deep physical/psychological insecurity, is that the further we went, the more lost I felt I was becoming, or might become, in the further reaches of 'darkest' Enfield. One thing was for sure; if Willow Walk was on the route, we were not going there directly. – After a brief detention in the police station at Edmonton Green, I was returned by panda car to Chase Farm. I willed the speeding car not to veer right onto the Ridgeway; ie, towards the hospital rather than homewards, but to no avail. The fact that one of the young officers reminded me facially

The Total Obliteration Of Hell

of the lead singer of the group 'Madness' gave me a faint hope that my wish would be granted, but I daresay that I was not altogether surprised when I did not get my way.

Frank Hayward

A love of objects

I referred under the heading 'Steve' to my attachment to the material things I'd accumulated at Willow Walk, and it is to this that I now turn.

The analogy that springs to mind when I think of the magnitude of the excitement I felt when in my room at home, both during my more successful escape attempts and later on whilst on leave (in 1987), is that I was like a child on Christmas morning, or at least, as I used to be as a child on the morning of December 25th, with a pillowcase full of presents to open and my loving family around me. Perhaps it is a testament to the degree of my mental disruption of 1987 that my possessions; particularly books that I had long been fond of, and perhaps even more particularly, anything and everything that I'd written myself, was/were able to arouse such emotion: - every text and piece of paper, whilst being familiar, seemed endowed with a beauty and intelligence far beyond anything I'd noticed before. And the sense of discovery was heightened by the fact that I didn't have much idea which drawer or cupboard currently housed my most prized books and writings; i.e., the thought that, since everything seemed special, then those things that I already considered of particular merit would seem even more so, had time to blossom before I managed to locate them. The anticipation was a tad frustrating, but I was excited to fever pitch, and my desperate searching would periodically exhume more 'treasure' although, once I'd found the item in

The Total Obliteration Of Hell

question, I'd put it down and promptly lose it again, there being so much clutter, and my mental processes being in such disarray. As regards my finds; Lola's letters, and my piece of writing entitled 'The World of Lola Jimenez Part 1', were undoubtedly amongst the items whose unearthing gave me the most complete satisfaction, but old holiday diaries; cassette tapes with recordings of my musical compositions; my Shirley MacLaine autobiographies, and my college dissertation on reptile conservation, all aroused ecstatic reactions in their turn. – So obsessed was I by the thought of the delight aroused in this way that I often imagined, when at the point of falling asleep in my hospital bed, that I could 'relocate myself' to my bedroom at home simply by wishing myself there. This 'trick' had a connection with a quite crazy idea I dreamed up for 'dealing with' a most singular patient who, whilst neither describable as friend or foe, produced a lasting impression on me.

Philip

My acquaintance (if even that word is not a euphemism in its implied suggestion of some sort of relationship) with Philip, began some time prior to my admission to hospital in 1987. I cannot remember for certain when I first became aware of this 'curious creature', but I think the location was the Day Hospital.

The word mad, when applied to the mentally ill, is very often entirely inappropriate, since it evokes an impression of total irrationality and alarming unpredictability; ie, when it is in fact usually the case that the behaviour of the 'average' mental patient shows much more conformity to a pattern than this implies. Indeed; when such factors as paranoia are taken into account, many 'mentally unbalanced' reactions to situations can actually seem quite rational. Perhaps this raises questions about the appropriateness of my having referred to myself as mad in these writings? However, whether it makes sense to describe my behaviour or state at this time as mad, my experience of the mentally ill inclines me to make an important distinction between those individuals whose behaviour is to a certain extent comprehensible, and with whom some meaningful communication is possible, and a much smaller category of those who, whilst being fully conscious and able to function 'normally' in many ways, are yet on such a different 'wavelength' as to be beyond understanding, and entirely (or very largely) incommunicable with. Whilst I would,

The Total Obliteration Of Hell

with some reservations, place my psychotic self in the former category, Philip was, and to the best of my knowledge still is, a 'person' whose condition makes him an obvious candidate for the second. (I have used inverted commas because 'person' (arguably) suggests personality, and I don't know that Philip can be said to have one any more than a willow tree can be said to possess personality because its branches creak in the wind.) But I am not intending to suggest that Philip, or any other 'person' describable as a member of this second category, is/are of less significance than other human beings. To illustrate the hopeless impossibility of relationship with 'individuals' such as Philip, I will make the following analogy. If, of three people, two share a common language, and the third does not know the language and speaks in a tongue that is alien to the other two, then the potential for relationship between the two is clearly greater than that between either of the two and the third person. And if a similar situation pertains in relation to other, non verbal forms of communication, there is no basis whatsoever for any relationship between that person and either of the other two. The 64,000 dollar question is whether the behaviour of such organisms as Philip is in fact rational in its own terms, and would be to whosoever unlocked the code that he/they use/s?

Loosely then, without simply seeking to sensationalize, Philip was (and I believe still is) quite mad as far as I was concerned, for I could not (and still cannot) understand a blind word he said, except when he asked me for cigarettes. (One might quite reasonably question my ability to have found meaning in Philip's behaviour bearing in mind the state that I was in. However, no one else appeared to understand him either.)

Whether Philip consciously tried to communicate his 'world view' to those around him, and whether he even recognized the existence of other conscious beings, it is not easy to be sure, but his demeanour; he was bearded, and there was an openness and purity in his face; and the manner in which he spoke; he was often intensely serious; conveyed the impression of a sage. I recall that another patient also felt that Philip was a very wise man, or at least that he gave a convincing impression of one. Another factor that helped to create the impression that Philip was special was the combination of the incomprehensibility of his words and the steely-eyed assurance with which he delivered them, and, coupled with this was the subject matter of his utterances, which seemed to concern suffering and torture, but were conveyed without complaint or self pity. Indeed, when he did mention 'himself', it tended to be only in the third person. – The impact on me of this diminutive figure, whose countenance could be as forbidding as my hero Clint's, was often to precipitate guilt and shame in me at my self concerns and ignorance of the 'universal truths' that he was expounding: - I sometimes felt that Philip was very subtly trying selflessly to point me towards enlightenment. And what did I do but patronize him and laugh at the way he walked and at some of his most commonly

The Total Obliteration Of Hell

used phrases such as 'left-hand side of shell', and 'Quentin Heman's left fist'!

My 'plan' for Philip was, as I reflect upon it now, rather sinister, in that it involved my taking on a God-like role, and could even be described as murder, since it necessitated 'doing away with' one person. However, the fusion of the minds of Philip and my mentally-handicapped brother Tim in order to create one embodied, 'competent' individual from two 'unfortunate' beings, was certainly something that I was at the time prepared to consider. Needless to add, the 'plan' was no more than this wish, and a belief that such a thing was possible, and (I think) that I could achieve the desired result simply by the force of my concentration, once I'd 'transported' Philip to Tim's bedroom at Willow Walk. My belief in the possibility of such a fusion of beings is rather similar to another notion that I had about what might loosely be called cloning although, as I will explain in the following chapter, this process, which I believed had commenced on a universal scale, was not just the duplication of unique individuals, but a phenomenon whose implications were far more alarming.

All personality/ies In jeopardy

I have already spoken at some length of my conviction whilst in hospital that certain 'hapless patients' and 'members of staff' were really only masquerading as such, and were in fact famous pop stars, actors, politicians etc; or at least, 'versions' of these famous people. The list of these celebrities, both living and deceased at that time (being deceased being no problem to me in terms of believing that I'd seen them) is lengthy, and includes not only those already mentioned; namely, John Lennon, Yoko Ono, Dustin Hoffman, Peter Gabriel and David Steele, but also Meryl Streep (a flaxen haired girl in the typing pool on the top floor in 1985), Andrew Ridgeley (one half of pop duo 'Wham'), Mahatma Gandhi, Gerald Durrell, Bruce Forsyth, and Harrison Ford, at whom I couldn't help giggling because he'd been considerably 'uglified'. There were also various assorted Shirleys and Clints, all of whom were decidedly poor versions of the original. And then of course, Anna 'was' Lola, and her husband 'was' my friend Robert Olivier; the list goes on.

However, my point here is not simply to enumerate, and paint thumbnail portraits of, the characters that I have not already described, but rather to endeavour to put across the sense in which I felt, particularly in 1987, that personalities (and not only those of celebrities), and the distinct appearance of individuals, were being whittled away, as if by a virus; 'divine retribution' for the extent to which

The Total Obliteration Of Hell

society 'had declined' into a dichotomy of media superstars (the celebrities of sport and show business) and a passive, characterless general population who lived vicariously through these larger than life 'demigods' of stadium and screen. I don't believe that I consciously thought in these terms at the time, but it did seem that no one, however big the name or strong the personality, had the ability to 'hold their soul together'.

So, what I sensed was happening was that, for example, Shirley MacLaine (as we know it!) was 'splitting' into a number of diluted versions of herself, and so was everyone else. I'm not sure whether I felt that it was possible that the original star or other person might remain in their own body, with their personality intact, but in a severely weakened form, horrified by the thought of what perverse things their 'clones' might be getting up to! – That such a thing might be happening was a dismal thought, but especially so when it concerned those who I had up to this point held most dear. However, the possibility that I might suffer a similar fate was perhaps a matter of more direct concern; after all, 'I was all I had'!, besides which, if I was the only person fully aware of what was happening, then it was vital that I should not lose myself before we all became vacillating, amorphous, passionless, soulless beings!

Frank Hayward

'Gelli'

I have mentioned Gelli briefly already under the heading 'The Weetabix', and in connection with my memories of Lincoln Ward, when I'd fancied that he was the actor Dustin Hoffman. And, in my deranged condition of 1987, I was once again quite ready to believe that, whether or not this was his true identity, he was at least a version or 'alter ego' of said famous individual. This impression was heightened, or possibly reactivated, when the Hoffman film 'Little Big Man' was shown on T.V. in the dayroom. I believe that I'm correct in saying that Gelli was present for at least part of the duration of this flick, and his animated reaction (as I remembered it) to what I assumed to be Dustin's presence on screen, either confirmed, or triggered off, my feeling of old.

I was very impressed by the athleticism and seeming bravery of Dustin's character in the film, and felt quite certain that he had really lived the part and was passionately respectful of American Indians, and I suppose that it would be true to say that I transferred these feelings of respect from the screen star to Gelli, who it seemed to me must also possess such courage and compassion for his fellow man. However, as the months slipped by, and Gelli remained as apparently lost and juvenile as ever, so I guess this reverence imperceptibly slipped away. It would probably be fair to describe Gelli as having been on 'another planet', much as Philip appeared to be. However, the extent of Gelli's displacement to another realm cannot I think compare with the total isolation of Phil' since, in Gelli's case, conversation was at times possible to a degree, and there was an occasional sense of 'togetherness' when sharing a joke that was never possible with young Philip.

Happy ever after?

By the time that my father died in June 1987, my 'alternative reality' had largely faded away, although I was left with a certain residual amount of misplaced enthusiasm. I don't believe that I was in the least bit traumatized by dad's passing, but I daresay that it might be suggested that my subsequent decline into a second period of depression during July of that year was probably related to his death. For the next 18 months or so I did very little apart from chain-smoke, and appreciated even less. At midnight on New Year's Eve 1989, whilst alone at Willow Walk, and far from eager at the prospect of a new decade, I made my only suicide attempt to date; pills and alcohol: - I was fortunate to avoid having my stomach pumped.

Curiously enough, although I am to this day adamant that death was my aim on that occasion, January 1990 did not prove to be 'beyond endurance', and, as the spring progressed, so I felt a certain sense of hope. I particularly associate this feeling with my efforts at pruning our apple trees. However, it was not until September 1991, when I followed the advice of Lena, my Community Psychiatric Nurse, and dared to return to camping/hillwalking that I really began to feel that life was worth living once again.

The Total Obliteration Of Hell

Concluding note

It is perhaps a foolish temptation, as someone who has enjoyed relatively good health for the past few years, to suggest that my episodes of illness have fulfilled a beneficial function, and even to go as far as to propose that such illnesses always occur for a good reason. However, although I am relatively certain that it is very dangerous to believe that the intensely disturbing experiences of such an affliction necessarily have a 'silver lining', I would dare to suggest that the potential for self realization through mental illness is tremendous, in that the shattering effect that it can have on one's idea of the world can act as a sort of purge, rather in the manner that frost, by breaking up the surface of soil, renders it more suitable for new growth. The limitations of this analogy are at once obvious, since the shattering effects of frost on soil can hardly be said to render it 'insane', and it is also (regrettably) all too often the case that the disorienting shock of a mental breakdown does not give way to 'rebirth' or new growth, but is succeeded only by trauma, depression, and, all too frequently, attempts to commit suicide. This begs the question why it is that some people recover whilst others continue to suffer on a more permanent basis? One answer would be that it has to do with an individual's karma; ie, to explain what happens in relation to past actions, both in this life and in 'previous incarnations'; - the resultant ease or difficulty of recovery thus being regarded as a consequence of past action. I must admit to feeling rather cagey about such an explanation, because it is all too easy to lose one's compassion for the suffering of others if all suffering is regarded as being one's 'just desserts', and because I don't really understand why different individuals should have established different karma assuming that we all started on an equal footing at the beginning of our 'first lifetime'.

Another question to which I cannot honestly claim to have any really satisfactory answer is perhaps a step back from the issue of recovery/lack of recovery; namely, why does mental illness 'select' the particular individuals it does? The received wisdom in contemporary mainstream psychiatry is that such conditions are caused by some or other traumatic life event or the disorienting effect of the abuse of alcohol or drugs triggering a genetic predisposition towards such conditions, a predisposition present in some individuals but not in others. But this is not a teleological explanation; ie, it merely attributes mental illness to a cause, and thus doesn't really explain its origin beyond it being a matter of chance or 'bad luck'. Maybe in truth there is no explanation beyond this, but for myself I am again inclined to invoke the possibility of karma. In relation to my personal experience I can perhaps be more specific, and would suggest a twofold explanation for my periods of insanity. Firstly, I was eager to question the nature of reality, and the illness was an opportunity to really go into it, and secondly, and rather similarly, I tended to challenge things, and to regard myself as almost impossibly clever, and the illness represented the 'fall'; ie, an inevitable consequence of my conceit and pride. However, if this implies that I now regard myself as being at a sort of 'advanced stage', and that I am now rid of ego, I hope that I would be the first to admit that that is far from true, and that I see no good reason to suppose that I am now somehow immune to further episodes of madness. But then, aren't you the reader also a potential candidate?

Lightning Source UK Ltd.
Milton Keynes UK
04 September 2009

143369UK00001B/10/P